CAREER DIRECTIONS

for

DENTAL HYGIENISTS

By

Regina A. Dreyer, RDH

Career Directions Press
171 Highway 34, Holmdel, New Jersey 07733

Career Directions for Dental Hygienists. Copyright 1987 by Regina A. Dreyer. Printed and bound in the United States of America. All rights reserved. No part of this book may be reproduced in any form or by any electronic or mechanical means including information storage and retrieval systems without permission in writing from the publisher, except by a reviewer who may quote brief passages in a review. Published by Career Directions Press, 171 Rte. 34, Holmdel, NJ 07733. Revised edition.

ISBN 0-933163-01-0

Library of Congress Catalog Card Number 87-071570

Cover design by Karen Forgash

Foreword

I am a dental hygienist. I started out as a dental hygienist. I am always proud to be a dental hygienist. These words remain true for me whenever I say them.

As I look back on my endeavors, I can see the intertwining of my entry skills in dental hygiene. President, director, administrator, faculty, board member—all have built upon my background. I am proud of my accomplishments but I do not feel I have reached the limits our profession has to offer.

Dental hygiene is our profession. What we do with our careers in it is based on the initial education we have received. We are always dental hygienists. Some of us have taken different paths and hold positions other than clinical dental hygiene. We have expanded our employment settings to include managers, administrators, public health workers, industrial researchers and sales personnel. Each role builds on the talents we have acquired as dental hygienists. Our profession is still expanding and its future shows many new promises.

There is no time for discussions of burnout or boredom. If frustration has set in, it is merely time to self-assess and plan for the future. It is not time to leave your profession behind. Let us consider career options in dental hygiene, not a change in careers.

As you read through the following chapters, I challenge you to think of the new roles for yourself in dental hygiene. These contributors will spark an excitement and renew your commitment for our profession. Set up your opportunities now and plan for your next success. Reach out with me as we explore *Career Directions for Dental Hygienists*.

Cheryl Westphal, RDH, MS, President
American Dental Hygienists' Association, 1984-85

Fairleigh Dickinson University, Director
Division of Dental Hygiene
Hackensack, New Jersey

To My Parents

Samuel and Esther Shear

Table of Contents

Introduction

Suppose you were at the beach and saw a lovely piece of colored glass lying half-buried in the sand. When the sun hit the part that wasn't covered, you were caught by the sparkle and picked up the glass.

Turning it over and over, you examined your find as the sunlight heightened and intensified the color. Only then did you realize how many facets there were, how many angles and surfaces made the glass whole and gave it its depth and radiance. The sparkle that caught your eye was not reflected from the whole piece, only one side of it.

Look at the profession of dental hygiene the same way. Are you seeing only one dimension? Are you caught up in boundaries that exist only because you're not looking at the other sides?

Opportunity, unlike the glass on the beach, is wherever you find it.

Dental hygienists from the beginning have always had the ability to move in and out of private practice environments into other arenas of health care, but never as easily and with as many choices as now.

I should know. Since getting my license over thirty years ago, I have been a school dental hygienist, private practice office manager, supervisor of a hospital-based public health program, clinical instructor in a school of dental hygiene, director of educational services for a dental manufacturer, writer. And always with RDH after my name.

Building professional experiences, acquiring degrees, having a family—all are part of a career pattern. And that is the philosophical focus of this book: dental hygiene is a *career,* not a series of jobs in one setting. Private practice is an *option*—not a locked room.

Through this book you will be introduced to over twenty dynamic, achieving RDHs who have taken their skills and abilities and parlayed them into a variety of experiences which are bringing them fulfillment and professional satisfaction. The kind of satisfaction that comes from accepting a challenge and mastering it.

Perhaps you know some of these dental hygienists. Or would like to know them, talk to them, share their pride in being a part of constructive change.

Their personal histories reveal compelling tales of growth. The authors are neither superwomen nor malcontents. Quite the contrary. Each one exhibits a unique, upbeat identity and an exhiliration for life, our profession, and the process of change.

If self-awareness is one of the keys to success, examine not only *how* these people achieved but *why*. What is it that motivates them? Why isn't what they're currently doing ever enough? Is it restlessness? Dissatisfaction? I think not. I think it is a never-ending curiosity about what else is out there "around the corner." They want to mesh opportunity with their personality needs. (See the first chapter which tells you how to assess *your* personality style.)

I can almost hear some of these writers saying (and though I've not met many of them, I feel as if I know them through their contributions), "What if. . .?" Or, after looking into something, "Hmm. I wonder . . . " Always questioning, always eager to see if and where a stone can be turned, another avenue explored.

See if you don't agree. See if you don't identify with many of their feelings. Listen to how they made their decisions. Hear how they conquered their fears and insecurities. The *process* is as exciting in its unfolding as is the achievement itself.

About the authors. Where did I find them? Mostly word of mouth starting with the ones who are my friends. This one knows that one and that one knows this one . . . And now, through this book, we know them all! With few editorial changes, the respective voices are as spoken. I am deeply grateful to each one of them for the care and thought that went into their writings. It made the book worthwhile.

I also owe considerable thanks to RDH general contributors Joan Babecki, Dorothy Fosket, Phyllis Janofsky, Rochelle Leyba, Patti Miller, Annette Scheive, Jan Shurts, Julie Yergler, and to the newest development in my career, my husband Neil Thomas.

In writing articles over the past several years (some of you may recognize my name from *RDH* magazine or as editor of my own newsletter), I've researched many arenas of health care. I have a file on health career management which I want to share with you.

Interwoven with the histories are my own contributions on various dental delivery systems, post-certificate degrees, government positions, tips on presenting yourself through your résumé, and other information you need to fine-tune your thinking about your career.

At the end of the book, I've included a resource list for obtaining specialized information on health care environments, programs, and delivery systems.

I wrote and edited *Career Directions for Dental Hygienists* because I believe the growth of our profession demands a resource devoted exclusively to career opportunities and their successful management. I hope that premise, reflected in the writings, meets your expectations and fills your needs in reaching your own career goals in dental hygiene.

Upward and onward!

Regina Dreyer, RDH
Editor & Publisher

Summer 1987

"THERE'S ONLY ONE CORNER OF THE UNIVERSE YOU CAN BE CERTAIN OF IMPROVING, AND THAT'S YOUR OWN SELF."
—Aldous Huxley

Personality Type
and
Career Choice

Denise M. Hart, Ed.D., Associate Professor

Dr. Denise Hart began her career in dental hygiene as a clinician in private practice and as a faculty member in a school of dental hygiene.

She has remained in the academic setting in a variety of educational roles, currently directing the Office of Adult Education for adult learners in the Colleges of Arts and Science and Liberal Arts at Fairleigh Dickinson University in New Jersey.

Her educational research reflects her commitment to dental hygiene as a sound base upon which to build personal and professional growth patterns. As she says, "I will always consider dental hygiene as my introduction to the socialization of people in a health care setting. What this means is having a deep concern about what your patients think and need, and being there to help them make a responsible decision for their own care."....

Personality Type and Career Choice: Match or Mismatch?

How would you describe yourself, most of the time? Are you practical or instinctive in your observations? Are your judgments made with personal or impersonal analysis?

Every individual is a composite of several traits which can identify an individual's personality type. Some people are very "true to type". In other words, they behave the same way a majority of the time under similar circumstances. These are people whose behavior and reactions can be anticipated.

In opposition, are those individuals whose perceptions and judgments are not clearcut and who may seem unpredictable. However, each individual has a preferred type and will probably always remain that type.

An individual's personality characteristics are unique to that person and inherent. One's interests, beliefs, values *and* accomplishments are based on the effective use of the strengths and weaknesses of the individual personality structure. Some traits will become more dominant during the course of normal development and will guide the individual's understanding and decision-making.

Determination of an Individual's Personality Type

Which characteristics are most like you? Place a check mark next to the statements that describe yourself *MOST OF THE TIME.* Total the number of check marks in each list. Utilize the column that has the highest number of check marks in each of the four sets of attributes to determine your personality profile. (A diagram for the personality preferences depicted in this exercise is found at the end of this chapter. Refer to it once you have *completed* the exercise. Do not cheat yourself by looking at the blueprint first.)

(First Set)

____At social gatherings, is comfortable at introducing themselves to other guests	✓ At social gatherings, needs to be introduced to other guests
✓ prefers to work in large groups and with a number of other individuals	____prefers to work alone, or with one or two other individuals only
____can work in a frenetic environment; not annoyed by interruptions	✓ prefers to work in a quiet place; annoyed by interruptions
✓ outspoken, shares personal experiences	____quiet, introspective
____dislikes complicated tasks, prefers to act quickly, sometimes without knowing all the facts	✓ prefers to work intently on a project, understanding it first, thoroughly prepared
_2_ total # of check marks	_3_ total # of check marks

(Second Set)

✓ down to earth, practical	____ethereal, possibility-thinker
✓ learns best by following sequential pattern, step-by-step	____learns best by "seeing" the whole picture

3

____needs to have clear-cut picture

____prefers memorizing and working with true facts

____enjoys routine

___✓_can see with the mind's eye

___✓_prefers interpretation and working with possibilities

___✓_enjoys new ways of doing things

_2_ total

_3_ total

(Third Set)

____impersonal, nonpartisan

____makes decisions based on logic, cause and effect

____able to reprimand, business-like

____more truthful than tactful, if forced to choose

___✓_likely to assert individual opinion rather than defer choice to others

___✓_personal, subjective

___✓_makes decisions based on personal values

___✓_dislikes telling people unpleasant things, avoids disharmony

___✓_more tactful than truthful, if forced to choose

____likely to agree with others in a group rather than assert an individual opinion

_1_ total

_4_ total

(Fourth Set)

___✓_lives by "shoulds" and "oughts"

___✓_likes plans, schedules

____may come to conclusions too quickly without considering all the aspects

____has a live and let-live attitude

____likes impromptu arrangements

____takes time in drawing conclusions, so much so that at times things may be left incomplete

4

___√___likes closure,   _____likes spontaneity
       finality

___√___prefers to work on one   _____may start many projects
       project at a time, may   simultaneously and have
       even ignore other   difficulty in completing
       matters in completion   them
       of project at hand

___ɥ___total   __|__total

(When you have reached this point refer to the diagram at the end of the chapter to determine your personality profile.)

Each individual's personality type is made up of four preferences: Extraversion or Introversion (E or I), Sensing or Intuition (S or N), Thinking or Feeling (T or F), and Judging or Perceiving (J or P). The composite is identified by four letters which represent the individual's preferences i.e., ESTJ, ENTJ, ISTJ, INTJ, etc. There are sixteen possible four-letter profiles.

Within the four-letter combination, the first letter represents an individual's orientation to life, whether they be interested in people and things (E) or ideas and concepts (I).

The second letter represents how an individual perceives or becomes aware, either through Sensing (S) where one utilizes the five senses; sight, sound, touch, taste, feel or; Intuition (I) where the individual relies on insight.

The third letter represents the means for making decisions based on what has been perceived, either through Thinking (T) where an individual judges by means of impersonal analysis or Feeling (F) where the individual relies more on subjectivity and personal values.

The fourth scale, Judging (J), Perceiving (P) defines the individual's behavior in the extraverted part of her life. The (J) individual prefers closure and advanced planning, while the (P) likes flexibility and spontaneity.

Each of the preferences points to an extreme. An individual is not all of one characteristic and none of the other; however, the stronger characteristics prevail and are relied upon.

A dominant type is represented by the individual's favorite of the two central preferences, Sensing and Intuition or Thinking and Feeling. Likewise, there is a "second-in-command", the auxiliary preference which is the complement within the two central preferences. If an individual's dominant preference is either S or N, then her auxiliary preference will be either T or F and vice versa.

5

It is the combination of the dominant and auxiliary types that assists the individual in determining learning styles and commitments, while the E-I scale points to one's natural interests and the J-P scale shows one's work habits.

Which job is best suited to my personality type?

Research has shown that particular combinations of the personality type preferences are associated with specific vocational choices. Below, is a chart excerpted from Isabel Briggs Meyers, *Manual, The Myers Briggs Type Indicator* (1962, p. 56) which displays the characteristics and job possibilities associated with the two central preferences.

	ST	SF	NF	NT
People who prefer:	SENSING + THINKING	SENSING + FEELING	INTUITION + FEELING	INTUITION + THINKING
focus their attention on:	Facts	Facts	Possibilities	Possibilities
and handle these with:	Impersonal analysis	Personal warmth	Personal warmth	Impersonal analysis
Thus they tend to become:	Practical and matter-of-fact	Sympathetic and friendly	Enthusiastic & insightful	Logical and ingenious
and find scope for their abilities in:	Technical skills with facts and objects	Practical help and services for people	Understanding & communicating with people	Theoretical & technical developments
for example:	Applied science Business Production Construction Etc.	Patient care Community Service Sales Teaching Etc.	Behavioral science Research Literature & Art Teaching Etc.	Physical science Research Management Forecasts & analysis Etc.

The dominant preference, since it is the one which sets the direction for your life as a whole, can direct the individual in making an educated career choice. Remember, the dominant function in one's personality is the individual's strongest link. In unison with the preference for Extraversion or Introversion, we can examine opportunities to earn a living within a milieu that has an ideal fit.

If your dominant preference is:

Extraverted Sensing - Look for an environment where you're among other individuals and working with your five senses.

Introverted Sensing - Look for an environment where you are using factual material but prefer to work alone or with a limited number of people.

Extraverted Intuition - Your job's most important feature should allow for creativity and continual challenge working with other individuals.

Introverted Intuition - Your best job utilizes your creativity and insight alone or in combination with a limited number of people.

Extraverted Thinking - Look for an environment which requires putting things in logical order without complicated step-by-step procedures.

Introverted Thinking - Your best job includes the ability to make decisions impersonally; contented to work alone, careful with details.

Extraverted Feeling - Most important is a harmonious relationship with others!

Introverted Feeling - Your job must make you feel good about yourself so that you can have inner peace.

Examine the following job categories. (These are limited in number and only an example. A complete list of occupations can be found in an occupational interest inventory.) Place a check mark next to those careers in which you are interested.

7

After you have completed this first step, go back and number these choices from one (1) to thirty-four (34) with *one* being your first choice. Then, take a separate sheet of paper and list all the ideas you personally have associated with those particular career choices. List benefits and deficits, working conditions associated with that job, and educational requirements.

___Clinical/Counseling
    Psychologist
___College Professor
___Political Scientist
___Sociologist
___Social Scientist
___Adult Education
    Teacher
___Group Worker
___Nurse, General Duty
___Rehabilitation
    Therapist
___School Counselor
___Social Worker
___Special Education
    Teacher
___Speech Therapist
___Dental Assistant
___Licensed Practical
    Nurse

___Experimental Psychologist
___Physician
___Psychiatrist
___Medical Technologist
___Nurse, Practitioner
___Physician Assistant
___Dramatist
___Editor
___Critic (Reviewer)
___Fashion Artist
___Furniture Designer
___Interior Designer
___Package Designer
___Set Designer
___Clothes Designer
___Minister/Priest/Rabbi
___Librarian
___Medical Record
___ Librarian
___Dental Hygienist

What you have created is a very general "career map." At your local library you can use your career map to examine your presumptions against the *Dictionary of Occupational Titles* for a more elaborate outline of job descriptors.

Individual personality types are magnetized to specific attributes associated with a given work environment. Even the "group" personality type within the immediate parameters of your job environment will influence your gratification and fulfillment. Choose carefully . . . but remember it is never too late to modify or change your first choice.

Work satisfaction and success likewise depend on the degree of match between one's personality type and vocation.

The following is an exercise in **Goal Setting** taken from *Becoming a Master Student* (1984, pp. 48-49). Give yourself at least an hour to complete it. Use it as a reminder of what you see yourself doing and how you intend to get there. Good Luck!

Part one: long-term goals

Long-term goals represent major targets in your life. What are your major educational and career goals? What about your personal relationships? Do you want to travel? What do you want to accomplish in your life? Do you want your life to make a statement? What is it?

Section A

The first part of the exercise is an eight-minute brainstorm. For eight minutes write down, as fast as you can, everything you think you want to do or be in your life. Leave no thought out. Don't worry about accuracy. The object is to generate as many ideas as possible. Use a separate sheet of paper for your brainstorm.

Section B

After you have completed Section A, spend the next eight minutes looking over your list. Think about what you wrote. Read the list aloud. Then select three goals that are most important to you.

Write these goals in space provided.

Goal 1

Goal 2

Goal 3

Part two: mid-term goals

Mid-term goals are objectives you can accomplish in two to five years. They include goals like completing a course of education or achieving a specific career level.

Part three: short-term goals

Short-term goals are the ones you can accomplish in a year or less. These goals are specific. They can include goals about specific courses, financial goals that include exact dollar amounts, or personal goals requiring action now or in the very near future.

Section C

Read aloud the three long-term goals you selected in Section B. Choose ONE long-term goal on which to focus your attention. Then brainstorm below a list of goals you might achieve in the next two to five years that would lead to the accomplishment of that one long-term goal. Spend eight minutes on this brainstorm. Remember, neatness doesn't count. Go for quantity.

Section D

Review your list of mid-term goals in Section C, then select three that you think would lead to the accomplishment of the long-term goal you picked. Allow yourself about five minutes for this part of the exercise.

Goal 1

Section E

Review your mid-term goals in Section D. Select one. In another eight-minute brainstorm, generate a list of goals you can reach in a year or less that will lead to the accomplishment of that mid-term goal. As always in a brainstorm, write down everything that comes to mind. Do not evaluate or judge. The more ideas you write down, the better.

Goal 2

Goal 3

Section F

Review your list of short-term goals in Section E. Then cross out any that seem inappropriate. The most effective brainstorms are conducted nonjudgmentally, so you might find some bizarre ideas on your list. That's fine. Now is the time to weed them out.

Next evaluate your short-term goals to determine which ones you can accomplish and are willing to accomplish. Select three of these and write them in the space provided.

Goal 1

Goal 2

Goal 3

Part four

Take a few minutes to reflect on all the goals you selected in Sections B, D and F during this process. Look for relationships. Think about what accomplishing these goals means to you. Think about how the process felt.

The more you practice, the more effective you will be at choosing goals that have meaning for you. You can repeat this exercise using the other long-term goals you generated, or create new ones. Use the process to make long-term goals real in the here and now.

Diagram for Determining an Individual's Personality Type

(First Set)	E	I
(Second Set)	S	N
(Third Set)	T	F
(Fourth Set)	J	P

References

Myers, I.B., *Manual, The Myers Briggs Type Indicator.* Consulting Psychologists Press, Inc., Palo Alto, CA., 1962.

Ellis, D.B., *Becoming a Master Student,* College Survival, Inc., Rapid City, SD, 1962.

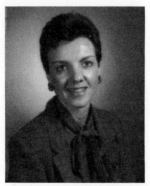

Dr. Denise Hart

RDH in Public Health

Introduction

Patricia Pretara Spanedda, *who worked as a dental hygienist in a community health setting, introduces this section on dental public health.*

One of Ms. Pretara Spanedda's major accomplishments was the initiation and implementation of a fluoride mouthrinse program in an urban community.

* * * * *

Today, career opportunities for the dental hygienist are numerous. One aspect of dental hygiene providing professional rewards, intellectual stimulation, personal creativity and job satisfaction is public or community health.

Public health is defined as "the science and art of preventing disease, prolonging life, and promoting health and efficiency through organized community efforts..."[1] Dental public health encompasses many phases of dental hygiene with emphasis on the educational and clinical services.[2] Prevention of disease, more specifically, dental caries, periodontal disease, cleft lip and cleft palate, and oral cancer is the primary goal of public health.[3]

Dental public health activities include public health education, school health education, nutritional counseling, child and adult care, "special needs" patient care, preventive measures, and collecting statistical data.

Methods of conducting these activities are through dental health education programs, outreach programs, surveys (screening and referral programs), fluoridation of water supplies, fluoride mouthrinse or tablet programs, clinical dental hygiene (sealants, oral prophylaxis, fluoride applications), community service (Children's Dental Health Week), and the development of materials and resources (handouts, pamphlets).

These activities often require dental hygienists to function as dental health educators, dental health resource people and/or dental hygiene administrators in nursing homes, schools, hospitals, resident homes, health departments, neighborhood health centers and dental schools.

Job descriptions for these positions vary according to the professional staff with whom one works and the target group receiving treatment or services.

Target populations are senior citizens, school children, handicapped citizens, teachers, parents, nurses, as well as other professional groups.

Specialized skills necessary for RDHs employed in public health positions include professionalism, good communication and writing abilities, leadership, enthusiasm and adaptability to different situations. Private practice experience and community or volunteer work can only enhance performance in a public health position.

If you desire to work as a dental hygienist in a community-based program, apply for an available position. How would you know where and when such an opening exists? Resources include your dental hygiene association, dental and dental hygiene journals, and dental and dental hygiene schools. You can achieve a system of networking by publicizing your interests, abilities and work experience to your college instructors, dental salespeople, and other dental hygienists and allied health professionals.

You might hear about a public health position in another state but are not able to relocate. Another way to obtain a local position is by creating one! For example, you'd like to work for your local health department but neither the position nor funds exist. Why not write a grant to fund, staff and initiate a comprehensive program of education, prevention and treatment for your community? If you're unfamiliar with grant writing, you can research the reference books in the public library and/or call the state department of health.

Grant proposals should include objectives, purposes, procedures, resources, budget, evaluation, summaries, references and your résumé. Be sure to gain the support of local and regional professional organizations (dental, medical, nursing, and other health professions).

Let's suppose you are presently employed as a clinical dental hygienist in a residential home for the handicapped and you want to expand your responsibilities and position to one of public health.

First, determine the need for dental health education among the residents and staff of the home. Research the number of residents receiving dental care at the clinic on a weekly/yearly basis, dental health practiced in the cottages, and the follow-up care given by the staff in the residents' cottages.

Approach the dental director, express your findings, expertise and desire to expand your position. That person's support is necessary. Then meet with the home's administrator and the dental director to present your proposal.

Your proposal should include your goals, the way you will implement the program, and the method of evaluating the success of your program. Once your proposal is approved, it will be your responsibility to be creative and use appropriate resources to justify the program's continuance.

The following histories will show you RDHs who have successfully demonstrated the process by which they shifted their career goals to community dental health programs.

References

[1]Hanlon, J.,   *Public Health Administration and Practice,* 6th ed. (St. Louis: The C.V. Mosby Company, 1974) p. 2-4.

[2]DePaola, D.P., and Cheney, S.G., *Preventive Dentistry* (Littleton, Massachusetts: PSG Publishing Company, 1979) p. 264-268.

[3]Ibid.

RDH in the Elementary Schools

Linda M. Buist *outlines her successful elementary school program as dental health educator.*

A New Beginning

After relinquishing my position in private practice, moving 2300 miles across the country to Arizona, and becoming a military wife, the idea of transitioning within the field of hygiene seemed in accordance with the nature of my life at the time. Here was my perfect opportunity to venture beyond cleaning teeth, just as I had ventured from my home.

This is not to imply that I have turned, or ever will turn, my back on clinical hygiene. On the contrary, I view clinical hygiene as the foundation of our profession, and place high value on maintaining clinical proficiency. I have in fact, maintained employment in private practice at all times since graduating as a hygienist seven years ago.

Thus, upon arrival in my new hometown, I initially sought, and obtained, a part-time position in private practice. This position not only gave me a foothold as a hygienist, but also gave me the opportunity to learn about the community of which I was now a part. What better means is there to learn about one's community than to obtain first-hand information from a wide variety of its members on a one-to-one basis? We can learn so much from our patients!

I soon discovered that I could continue my education here in town through an off-campus program offered by one of the state's universities. In the first course I took, I met a classmate who was a nurse at one of the local elementary schools.

One year prior to this time, I had been involved with teaching a course in community dentistry, which included the study of school dental programs for elementary students. Since then, I had become intrigued with the idea of working as a school hygienist.

When I met this nurse, I was reminded of the role of the school nurse in implementing health education programs for students. I expressed to her my interest in teaching dental health in the schools. To my surprise, she informed me of a dental health program which had just recently been initiated in her district. Furthermore, I was told that the hygienist administering the program would be leaving at the end of the school year. I decided to investigate.

19

What Was Needed

Qualifications and experience required for the position included dental hygiene licensure in the state of Arizona, a minimum of two years' experience as a dental hygienist (preferably with involvement in dental health education), and the ability to establish and maintain working relationships with teachers and nurses, and, of course, to relate well to children. It was recommended that educational preparation should include health education courses and methods of teaching health. In addition, the prospective employee was required to possess adequate knowledge of public health laws and programs.

Through my contact with the school nurse, I was able to meet with the hygienist and learn more about the Yuma Dental Health Program. I applied for the job before a position opening was ever announced, so I really had no competition.

I had secured an Arizona hygiene license prior to moving West, and had worked as a hygienist for nearly five years prior to applying for the public health position. I have always enjoyed working with children, and was now eager to collaborate with teachers and nurses to work with them in a school setting.

My formal education had led to an A.A.S. degree in Dental Hygiene and a B.S. degree in Allied Health Education. This had included completion of the health education courses recommended as appropriate preparation for the job. Because the community dentistry course I had taught included study of public health laws and programs, I had maintained competence in that area. By the beginning of the next school year, the position of dental health educator was mine!

The current salary range for full-time employment is $13,550-18,854 annually for ten months of service, starting at entry level, plus medical insurance and an undesignated amount of money for reimbursement for travel. Depending on availability of funds, other fringe benefits may include reimbursement for uniforms, conference meals, and continuing education.

The Program Itself

The four main components of the dental program are:
1) Fluoride "Swish 'n Spit" mouthrinsing;
2) Dental health curriculum and resources for teachers;
3) Classroom visits/oral hygiene instruction;
4) Dental screenings.

Nos. 2 and 3 above together comprise the education component of the program which has been my main area of concentration as dental health educator.

Fluoride mouthrinsing was initiated in Yuma on a limited basis in 1978 by the State Bureau of Dental Health. Public health hygienists from the Bureau conducted DMF (decayed, missing, and filled teeth) surveys on students of participating schools in an effort to document the effectiveness of the fluoride.

In the fall of 1981, the Bureau coordinated with a non-profit foundation which agreed to provide funding to increase the number of schools participating. They also agreed to employ a dental hygienist to provide preventive activities and educational programs for elementary students and teachers. The hygienist works under supervision of and in cooperation with local and state dental groups, including the Bureau. Supporting funds were provided by a local private corporation.

During the 1981-82 school year, the number of schools participating in fluoride mouthrinsing increased. Dental health curriculum was introduced to kindergarten through third grade (K-3) teachers of eight schools, and oral hygiene instruction was provided for participating K-3 classrooms by means of classroom visits by the dental hygienist.

I began my work as dental health educator in the fall of 1982. The fluoride mouthrinsing component continued to expand both geographically and numerically and now includes eighteen schools and approximately 9,000 students and teachers across Yuma County. In most schools, grades K-6 participate in the fluoride component.

Parental consent forms are obtained for new fluoride participants, and swishing begins in the fall. Much of the preparation for swishing is carried out by the school nurses, with teacher supervision in the classrooms. Nurses are provided with enough supplies for students to swish once weekly throughout the school year with the 0.2% sodium fluoride solution. The time involved in an average classroom is about five minutes. Studies of school-based fluoride mouthrinsing such as this have shown a reduction in tooth decay of up to 35-50%.

Dental health curriculum is provided for and explained to teachers of participating classrooms at faculty in-services. Each year, I meet with the teachers of those classrooms new to the program to introduce them to the program and curriculum. During my first year with the program, I also met with teachers who were second-year participants, to review curriculum materials and introduce new materials as necessary.

All teachers participating in the program are provided with appropriate lesson materials to teach four dental lessons to their students during the school year. Lessons include such topics as plaque, nutrition, parts of a tooth, the process of decay, and tooth safety. Pre- and post-testing may also be conducted to help determine the effectiveness of the education component.

Additionally, I visit approximately 160 of the classrooms each year to provide oral hygiene instruction. Those classrooms which are new to the program are prioritized over continuing classrooms, and K-3 classrooms are prioritized over the higher grades. As the number of participating classrooms continues to increase to full potential, classroom visits may be offered to alternate grades of each school in an attempt to provide uniform services for all schools in the county.

Classroom Techniques

All students are given a new toothbrush, and proper toothbrushing techniques are introduced or reviewed in each classroom. During my visit, I provide brushing instruction, in which each student brushes his or her teeth in the classroom without the use of toothpaste (dry-brushing). Because a limited amount of plaque on tooth surfaces will maximize the effectiveness of rinsing with fluoride, teachers are asked to store the toothbrushes in their classrooms and repeat the dry-brushing session once each week, just prior to the rinsing exercises. Parental letters are sent home with the students to reinforce the importance of proper dental care for their children.

In the younger grades, I also demonstrate, with the help of a student volunteer, what it is like to visit the dentist. Disclosing is demonstrated in the third grades, and flossing is practiced in the fourth to sixth grades visited.

The fourth component, dental screenings, consists of DMF surveys and dental inspections. All screenings involve limited examinations, utilizing only mirrors, explorers, and available lighting.

Evaluation Surveys and Screenings

DMF surveys are conducted to provide data for the State Bureau of Dental Health to document the effectiveness of the fluoride mouthrinsing exercises, and to help determine the oral health status of students in the Yuma area.

DMF surveys involve a tooth-by-tooth examination of individual students. Each tooth is recorded as either decayed, missing, filled, or normal. Baseline data is obtained on students of schools new to the program, and conclusive data is obtained at these schools some years later.

Dental inspections involve a less comprehensive examination. They are conducted basically to inform parents as to whether or not decay is visible in their child's mouth. Recordings are not made for each individual tooth.

As previously stated, public health hygienists from the Bureau conducted initial DMF surveys on the students of participating schools in 1978. In the 1982-83 school year, I conducted initial DMF surveys and dental inspections of nearly 1700 students of varying grades at the schools new to the program.

The screenings are coordinated with the nurse of each school, and arrangements are made for a volunteer to act as recorder. The location of the screenings is usually the nurse's office, but other rooms could serve as well. Only those students of even grades (K, 2, and 4) are surveyed for statistical documentation.

All students screened, whether or not DMF data is collected, are given a letter to take home to their parents. This letter indicates the general condition of the child's mouth. Where decay is apparent, parents are advised to seek dental care for their child. In some cases, where severe dental problems are identified, parents are notified by telephone in addition to the written report.

Community Activities

Along with the aforementioned activities, I have responded to special requests of other educators in the community. For example, I participated in "Career Day" activities at a local junior high school, and spoke to the "Introduction to Health Occupations" students at two local high schools. I also met with the members of the local dental society to maintain communication with them about the activities of the program and to seek input from them regarding future activities.

I have found my work as a dental health educator in the elementary school system to be both enjoyable and rewarding. The spontaneity of children is refreshing, and the level of cooperation of nurses and teachers is encouraging. Of greater significance however, is the fact that the work is necessary. When I present a child with a toothbrush at school and it is his or her first toothbrush, or when I observe the stubs of decayed teeth in a child's mouth, I realize that we have only begun to meet the needs before us.

For those hygienists interested in obtaining a position in public health, I would encourage you to seek possible openings. It is not necessary to terminate your current job or to relocate as I did. It is important, however, to aggressively *approach* the opportunity rather than to wait for the opportunity to come your way.

To learn "what's out there" in your community, expose yourself to other professionals. Attend continuing education seminars and/or hygiene association meetings, continue your formal education, subscribe to hygiene magazines and newsletters. Stay abreast. Focus on your strengths rather than on your limitations.

I value the knowledge and experience I have gained by working as a dental health educator. And, as my interests change, I hope to expand my knowledge and explore different areas within the dental field in an attempt to prepare myself for new opportunities. I am excited about those career possibilities which lie ahead for us as dental hygiene professionals!

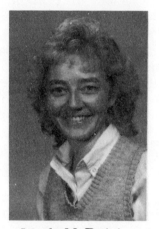

Linda M. Buist

*[Linda Buist would welcome comments or questions from interested readers. Contact her through **Career Directions Press**.]*

RDH in a Hospital

Mary Ann Curcio Piotrowski *discusses her personal and professional growth in hospital dental care programs.*

I can't believe the twist my career has taken! After working in middle management in a hospital setting for the last five years, I'm finally getting back to the basics—clinical dental hygiene. And in the same facility!

I've always loved hospital dentistry. Something exciting is always brewing.

What a Hospital Dental Center Is

Hospital dental centers are generally connected with general practice dental residency programs. These programs can be compared to medical internships except they are shorter in duration and completely optional.

Residency programs give new dental graduates an opportunity to expand their horizons and broaden their skills while treating patients with a wide variety of special needs.

Hospital dentistry is not for the squeamish or overly sensitive. Many of the patients are medically compromised with severe physical or mental handicaps, are victims of trauma, head and neck cancer, or carriers of infectious diseases. But to work in such an environment is a dynamic learning experience.

How I Got into It

I began working in a New York hospital as a dental assistant while attending hygiene school at night. Yes, I attended the only evening dental hygiene program in the country, the State University of New York at Farmingdale.

It took me a total of five years to complete the program: two years of prerequisites and three years of hygiene requirements. I had quite a hectic schedule what with holding down a full-time job and attending classes four nights a week until eleven o'clock!

I earned my degree the hard way. In retrospect, though, being an evening student made me a more disciplined person with added determination to reach success and achieve the goals I had set for myself.

25

Entering Supervision

While I was in school, the position of clinic supervisor opened up in the dental center. I really wanted that job and knew that I would be well suited for it. Fortunately, the director and clinic manager agreed. They were both familiar with my performance and the fact that I was continuing my education in dentistry enhanced my qualifications.

This position came with many responsibilities. Suddenly, I was accountable for the performance of employees and the daily operations of a busy dental clinic. I supervised the auxiliary staff and the dental residents; I was responsible for inventory control and the ordering of supplies; I was handyman. (To save time when equipment broke down, I usually tried to repair it myself before calling a serviceman.) I became a facilitator with one goal: to assure the quality of patient care.

When I became a hygienist, I decided to remain as clinic supervisor because I absolutely loved my job. Although I could have made a higher salary working in private practice, the hospital offered benefits that a dental office could not provide. These included stable hours with evenings and weekends free, all medical and dental insurance fully paid for, a life insurance policy and pension plan, a tuition reimbursement plan. In fact, the last two years of my hygiene education were paid for by the hospital. Not to be dismissed was the annual four-week paid vacation!

Moving into Middle Management

The biggest change to becoming an RDH came from the added respect I got from attending staff, dental residents, auxiliaries and the patients. I could legitimately discuss proper patient care in relation to departmental policy now because I was considered a colleague and co-therapist. I could develop protocol that would enable us to treat patients with special needs.

Patients with Infectious Disease

The hospital I worked in had the largest outpatient kidney dialysis center in the city. These dialysis patients were often Hepatitis B carriers. Being situated in New York City, many AIDS victims also sought dental treatment at our facility. Private practice environments are usually not prepared to treat carriers of such deadly diseases, and dental treatment in a hospital clinic is often their only hope.

Working closely with an infection control nurse, I developed specific guidelines for the isolation technique necessary to render proper treatment for these patients. My role then quickly changed to educator as I trained and oriented the entire staff to these new procedures. How proud I was when this project was successful!

Changing Jobs

When a change in my personal life forced me to leave my job and move to Philadelphia, I was excited and terrified at the same time. I love hospital dentistry, but I knew my chances of finding another position similar to the one I held were scarce. Even hospital positions in clinical dental hygiene are few and far between. Realistically I knew I would probably end up working in a private practice, but I was not totally resigned to the idea.

Then my lucky break came. I saw an ad in the Philadelphia paper for a dental clinic supervisor. Armed with my résumé, experience, and tons of enthusiasm, I interviewed for the position at Albert Einstein Medical Center—and got it. (To give you an idea how rare these positions are, the person I replaced had been working there for the last ten years.)

The program at Einstein consists of general practice, endodontic and orthodontic residency programs. When I started, the center was located in a very small area with old equipment. I was told that in the next six months the dental center would relocate and expand to a 21-chair facility with the latest in state-of-the-art equipment. The move would be complicated and the administrators were depending on me for some practical help and advice.

Gettings Things Done

I initiated many positive changes in the newly-expanded clinic. One of the most challenging problems concerned staffing. How was I to cover all areas of this enlarged facility with the same number of assistants?

Being in middle management really means *middle.* I bring my ideas for change to the manager and director and plead for their approval. If they agree, I issue a directive to my staff. Often staff is resistant to change and will express inward and outward disapproval. I've learned to deal with that. Middle management is not a position for someone who needs to be liked by everyone at all times.

There is a lot of red tape in any institution and a hospital is no different. For example, I need to get three signatures on a requisition for supplies before they can be ordered. Certain steps must be followed and change does come slowly. For a person who likes to have things done yesterday, this kind of situation can be frustrating.

Moving On

After two years, I felt that I had reached my potential in middle management. Although I had been attending evening classes, I did not yet have my bachelor's degree. The prospect of climbing up the management ladder was not realistic just yet. What's my next career move?

It was at this time that some significant developments occurred within the department. There had always been a part-time hygienist but the position had been vacant for almost a year. Approval was finally given for a full-time hygienist.

After much consideration, I applied for this position and was accepted. What an opportunity, I thought. I'll have the chance to create a full-time hygiene position in a hospital. And my salary will increase approximately five thousand dollars, too!

Since I had also been practicing hygiene part-time in a private practice, I was fully confident of my clinical abilities. I welcomed the shift in my job focus and the chance to communicate with patients on a more personal level. I looked forward to building my role as educator.

What I Currently Do

Some of the responsibilities of my new position include providing in-house education to various nursing units, developing a much-needed recall system, and working closely with the chairmen of periodontics and orthodontics to facilitate treatment of patients in these two areas.

Shortly I will begin treatment of hospitalized patients at their bedsides and participate in the Quality Assurance Program. The QAP is vitally important to the hospital because accreditation is largely based on the assurance of quality care.

If such work appeals to you, let the right people in the hospital know. Visit a dental center with yor résumé. Offer to volunteer some of your personal time there. Be positive and persistent. People will be impressed with your attitude and abilities. And who knows? *Your* name might pop into their heads when an opening *does* arise.

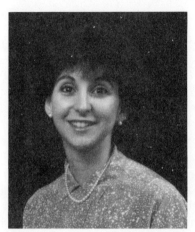

Mary Ann Curcio Piotrowski

29

In State Government

Ann M. Busch *has formed her career and professional goals as a consultant within the structure of state-sponsored programs in dental public health.*

My interest in dental public health began while I was enrolled in my associate degree program. I had an immediate interest in the community dental health course which was part of the overall dental hygiene curriculum. Visiting schools and developing and conducting community programs provided me with the variety I felt was lacking in clinical practice. I enjoyed all aspects of my schooling, but somehow I knew I wanted to learn more about the field of dental public health.

I inquired as to the additional training I would need to work in this field. My instructor was immediately supportive and encouraged me to apply to the bachelor's degree program, since a baccalaureate was a prerequisite. I was fortunate to be accepted the fall after graduation and looked forward to moving to the capitol city to be near the dental school.

A New Direction

During this school year, I had the opportunity to work independently on various community projects. I also found time to study further the subjects touched on during my associate degree years.

One particular assignment we were given was to work through the process of fluoridating a community water supply. Assistance for this project was available from the Indiana State Board of Health. I found this task exciting—from making contacts with local dentists—to hearing the votes come in, one by one, in *favor* of fluoridation!

Shortly after the completion of this project, I was made aware of possible job opportunities with the same health department. Each summer this State Board of Health hires hygienists and dentists to work with the migrant population in the state for the provision of basic preventive services. My classmate and I both applied and were accepted for the program that summer.

Working with migrant children and their families is a special public health offering of many state health departments. In our case, we enjoyed traveling throughout the state, educating the children, most of whom were bilingual, and providing a greatly needed service to this underprivileged group.

The summer soon came to an end. A full-time position was opening at the Indiana Board of Health. I have to say, it was a case of being in the right place at the right time. I have been in my current position for nearly five years and am enjoying it more than ever. I find this field of dental hygiene very rewarding both personally and professionally.

Variety—the Spice of Life

Each day of my week is in a different setting with new people and new challenges. I will never forget the day we screened prisoners' teeth in the state penitentiary, yet the very next day were sponsors of a large corporate health fair educating adults about good dental health! Ah, yes; variety.

My current responsibilities include school programs at all levels throughout the state which focus on dental health education and screenings. Weekly fluoride mouthrinse programs are promoted in cooperation with the university dental school. I've also initiated a fluoride supplement program for rural families through local indigent care clinics.

Another challenging project I've worked on is the production of a statewide telecommunications program for dental professionals. This means of providing continuing education through the university network system may someday become an annual event.

I now know I can be as creative as I want in this career and get as much out of it as I choose. At times I find it hard to push myself, but when I see the end to my means, I find the energy to continue. I'm a hard worker by nature and I sometimes find it hard to limit myself. However, I have learned that the enjoyment of my work comes from pushing myself to my fullest potential.

Working Together

My work in public health has enabled me to work with hundreds of other organizations and groups. This particular aspect enhances my satisfaction with my career choice. You have to want to jump right into your work and enjoy being involved. If, as a group, we cannot be excited about our profession and the things we stand for, we cannot expect the public to be either.

31

Involvement in my professional association at both the local and state levels has also served to help me further my career. I believe that however large or small, we all have something to contribute to our professional association.

Finally, submission of articles for publication is another means by which I feel a sense of reward. An article published about one of our programs or events helps me to see what I have done in black and white. Somehow, this serves as a reminder that I am making an impact with my efforts toward better dental health for the public.

Financial Rewards

I often hear of hygienists who hesitate about working in public health or government agencies because of low remuneration. I have found that my salary range is well within that of hygienists in private practice in my state, especially when I take into account the generous fringe benefits I receive. My current position allows for paid vacation, sick days, holidays, medical, dental and life insurance, and a retirement plan. Opportunities for attendance at professional meetings and continuing education programs are additional "perks" to this job.

As I write this synopsis of my career in community dental health, I am packing my bags to take on a new adventure. I have been accepted by another state health department to work with their migrant program for the summer. I am looking forward to experiencing the people, places and job responsibilities in a program where it all began for me.

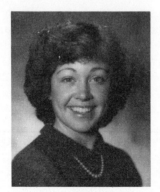

Ann Busch

*[Interested readers can contact Ann Busch through **Career Directions Press**.]*

Dental Hygiene Jobs in the Federal Service

What Do You Earn Working for Uncle Sam—and Where Are the Jobs?

Do you know who our nation's largest employer is? It's Uncle Sam, with 2.9 million workers (not including military personnel) on his payroll. If such employment interests you, consider this: there are approximately 385 full-time RDH positions in five federal agencies, the majority of which are in structured care settings such as hospitals and outpatient clinics.

The title "Dental Hygienist" is used for all positions primarily involving work of a clinical nature, including positions assigned duties related to research, teaching, or the performance of dental hygiene expanded functions.

Some 26 RDHs work in nonclinical settings assisting communities in planning and conducting dental health programs commensurate with the needs of the community. Their title, "Community Dental Hygienist" authorizes them for positions which are primarily nonclinical in nature and involve the planning, administration and evaluation of preventive oral health programs.

Most of these Community Health Dental Hygienists are with the Department of the Army, working throughout various large military installations. A few are employed by the Indian Health Service (Department of Health and Human Services). These positions are not only few in number but have a low turnover rate. It would be better for an individual interested in entering the Federal service to consider the position of clinical dental hygienist.

Which Five Agencies?

The Veterans Administration (VA) employs approximately 145 RDHs; the Department of the Army is next in staffing requirements being the largest of the Uniformed Services which also includes the Department of the Navy and the Department of the Air Force. (See list at end of book for names and addresses.)

Promotion potential is said to be good in the Department of the Army in their various military installations nationwide. The Air Force and Navy have far fewer positions and those only in hospitals.

On the Job Performance

What this translates into is that many dental hygienists in the Federal service are performing (under the direct supervision of a dentist) root planing, soft tissue curettage, administering infiltration anesthesia, in addition to planning dental hygiene treatment, assessing needs of patients, conducting oral health education on an individual and/or group basis not only in the clinic or hospital but outside the clinical setting. Bear in mind that the emphasis in the Federal service is on hospital dentistry.

Who Can Apply for Jobs—And Where?

The good news is that the qualification requirements for RDHs in the Federal service are the same as for the private sector: a license to practice from any state, territory or the District of Columbia. Obviously, the amount of knowledge required for a particular position, given the complexity, the scope, demands and the responsibilities of the assigned duties will be factors dictating grade level, and, by extension, salary. (More on duties a bit later.)

The bad news is that there is no centralized clearinghouse through which the positions are funneled. So how do you know if, where and when there are openings?

Since Office of Personnel Management (OPM) Regions are individually responsible for establishing and maintaining registers for clinical dental hygiene positions, start with your local Federal Job Information Center (FJIC). *There are no separate registers for Community Health Dental Hygiene positions. These positions are filled through special screening of qualified applicants for clinical positions.*

FJICs: What They Are and Where You Find Them

The OPM operates FJICs in all states, and often in more than one city in each state. They will be listed in your telephone book under "U.S. Government" or you can refer to the list in the back of the book.

The purpose of these centers is to provide general information on federal employment, explain how to apply for specific jobs and supply application materials. You can get information by mail, telephone, or by visiting one. Many FJICs also post state openings as well as Federal ones.

Salaries and Duties

The salary range for RDHs is from $14,822 for *Step 1* of the entry level GS-5, to over $22,000 for whichever *Step* you qualify for as a GS-9, the highest level assigned. Plus, of course, all benefits that Federal employees get. (Figures are for 1987 and can change.)

Most jobs posted seem to be in the GS-5 to GS-7 grade levels. Here are OPM benchmark descriptions for the duties of the GS-5, GS-6 and GS-7 positions. (Taken from the OPM's *Position-Classification Standard for Dental Hygiene Series GS-682*, TS-61, March 1982.)

Dental Hygienist, GS-5

Duties

Serves as a dental hygienist responsible for administering oral prophylaxis, treating abnormal gum conditions, and instructing patients in oral health care.

— Performs complete oral prophylaxis including the following: seats and drapes patients; applies disclosing solution to the teeth; performs supragingival and subgingival scaling using cavitron and scalers to remove calculus deposits, accretions, and stains; polishes teeth using bristle brushes, rubber cups, polishing strips, and prophylactic paste; and applies topical fluorides and other anticariogenic agents. Cleans and polishes removable dental appliances worn by patients.

— Examines patient's oral cavity including the mouth, throat, and pharnyx, and records condition of the teeth and surrounding tissues. Refers patients to the dentist who have abnormalities such as cavities, defective fillings, suspicious growths, or periodontal disease. Applies desensitizing agents and other topical agents to treat abnormalities such as gingivitis and Vincent's infection.

— Instructs patients, individually and in groups, in proper oral hygiene care using materials such as teeth models, displays, slides, toothbrushes, dental floss, disclosing tablets, mirrors, and phase microscope. Demonstrates proper techniques of brushing, flossing, and use of necessary perio aids and explains the common causes of tooth decay and its relationship to general diet. Instructs patients on the care of removable dental appliances. Instructs nurses and nursing assistants in oral health care techniques for bedridden, handicapped, disabled, and chronically ill patients.

— Takes, develops, and mounts oral X-rays including bite wing, panoramic and periapical. Interprets X-rays to determine areas of calculus deposits and periodontal involvement, the relationship of the teeth, etc. Selects and arranges X-rays as teaching devices for viewing by patients.

— Records the number of patients treated and type of treatment administered. Checks and maintains instruments to insure working condition. Cleans, sharpens, and sterilizes instruments.

Dental Hygienist, GS-6

Duties

Serves as a dental hygienist responsible for providing routine and advanced prophylactic and therapeutic dental care to postsurgical and periodontal patients.

— Upon referral from the dentist, examines patient's teeth and surrounding tissues to determine extent of abnormal condition requiring treatment. Records a history of each patient to determine if systemic conditions are present which may alter standard treatment. Plans dental hygiene treatment and series of appointments in accordance with existing conditions.

— Performs oral prophylaxis and provides therapeutic care in cases of acute gingivitis and periodontal disease using a variety of scalers and ultrasound equipment. Applies prescribed medicines to gums in cases of excess bleeding. When necessary, under the direction and supervision of the dentist performs deep scaling, root planing and subgingival curettage; takes intraoral impressions for the preparation of study models, smooths and polishes rough edges of restorations; places temporary fillings, administers local anesthesia; and places and removes rubber dams.

— In cases of periodontal surgery performs dressing removal, suture removal, irrigation, and dressing application. Provides therapeutic instruction to patient in the home care phase of treatment adapting instructions, oral hygiene aids and techniques to the individual situation. Teaches patients specialized techniques such as use of interproximal brushes, bridge threaders, and disclosing agents.

— Sets up and maintains a patient recall system to insure continuous, close follow-up treatment for each patient involved in the dental program. Provides instructions using demonstrations and audio-visual aids in the use and care of dental prosthesis, nutritional guidance, and need for daily hygiene care to prevent further dental disease and infections.

— Takes, develops and interprets intraoral and extraoral X-rays to determine areas of calculus deposits and periodontal involvement. Selects and arranges X-rays for special use in educating and motivating the patient.

— Provides dental hygiene instruction and training to other dental service personnel and participates in dental staff meetings and programs.

37

Dental Hygienist, GS-7

Duties

Serves as a dental hygienist responsible for performing advanced prophylactic and preventive dental procedures in the treatment of patients with related medical and dental problems.

— Completes preliminary dental examinations on new dental service patients. The hygienist reviews patient's medical and dental history for evidences of past and present conditions such as medical illnesses and use of drugs which may complicate or alter dental hygiene treatment; examines the teeth and surrounding tissues for evidences of plaque and periodontal disease and charts findings; inspects the mouth and throat for evidence of disease such as oral cancer; interprets routine X-rays to identify tooth structures, calculus, and abnormalities such as cavities and deep periodontal pockets. Refers abnormalities such as cavities, traumatic occlusion, and suspicious lesions to the dentist. Prepares dental hygiene treatment plans for patient including assessment of the problem, type of oral hygiene care required, and the sequence of appointments needed to complete treatment.

— Performs a complete oral prophylaxis on ambulatory and nonambulatory patients. Performs deep subgingival scaling, root planing, and curettage under local anesthesia. Polishes the teeth and applies stannous fluoride for hypersensitivity and caries prevention. Gives home care instructions to patients after curettage. Provides bedside prophylactic treatment using specialized procedures for comatose patients, neurosurgical patients, and other types of nonambulatory patients.

— In postoperative care of oral surgery and periodontal surgery patients, performs suture removal, changes dressings, applies topical anesthetics, and provides home care instructions. In oral cancer patients, takes impressions for construction of mouth guards, applies fluoride using tray technique, and maintains recall system for careful follow-up of each patient. Educates patient on need for daily oral health and fluoride treatment.

— Assists the dentist by making repairs and adjustments to the teeth by smoothing rough edges of restorations, removing overhanging margins of fillings, reducing sharp edges of fractured teeth, polishing and finishing amalgam restorations, and inserting temporary fillings in teeth.

— Instructs patients at chairside in oral hygiene, brushing and flossing techniques, and periodontal aids which increase the amount of stimulation to the teeth. Plans and adapts instructions in home care techniques, tailoring them to the oral hygiene needs and oral problems of individual patients. Explains to patients the causes of periodontal disease and tooth decay, and the importance of diet as it relates to oral and systemic health.

— Regularly instructs nurses and nursing assistants in the proper techniques of oral hygiene to be applied to the bedridden, handicapped, disabled and chronically ill patient. Presents lectures and demonstrations in oral health care to various patient groups such as diabetics, hemodialysis patients, and drug or alcohol dependent patients, using slides, denture models, toothbrushes, charts, and other dental education materials.

— Exposes, develops and processes radiographs on patients including bite wing, periapical and panoramic X-rays. Adjusts voltage, amperage, and timing of X-ray equipment. Selects type of radiograph that will be necessary for patient's mouth. Positions film and machine to insure coverage of area to be X-rayed. Mounts and labels X-rays.

— Maintains patient's record of treatment. Records oral conditions of the teeth and surrounding tissues, progress and therapy notes, appointments, and the number of patients treated and type of treatment administered.

Other Approaches

In addition to visiting the FJICs, you can do your own research. Call or write the chief dental officer of a VA hospital, Department of the Army military installation (remember, those two agencies employ the majority of the 385 positions), Department of the Navy or Department of the Air Force.

Ask if they employ RDHs at that facility, and, if so, do they anticipate any openings in the near future. What you don't want to do is send your résumé just on the chance there might be an opening. They don't file applications for unadvertised positions. The office of the chief dental officer is your best starting point for information.

Federal Prisons

Depending on Federal budgets, opportunities for RDHs open up from time to time in Federal prisons. Although these correctional institutions are under the Department of Justice, each institution hires contract personnel according to its individual budgets. Many budgets allow for a permanent full-time or permanent part-time dental hygienist. If so, the job is usually advertised in the local newspaper.

Unlike other Federal agencies which do not maintain registers, it is possible for you to contact the chief dental officer of an individual facility and ask that your name be kept on file in the event that a position becomes available. The advantage of doing this is that you are in a visible spot *before* the job is advertised.

If such a job would interest you, look under "US Gov't." in the telephone book for the names and locations of the prisons. (Not every state has them.)

A Government Careerist

Consider Joan Babecki who has developed her career within a VA hospital, beginning as a staff hygienist.

For her starting position on the GS-6 level, the requirements were either a bachelor's degree and three years' experience (plus, of course, licensure) or, as was Joan's case, an associate's degree with five years' experience.

Now, 12 years later, Joan reports, "I recently completed 186 hours of continuing education in a government-sponsored expanded functions program. This advanced training not only qualifies me to perform other clinical tasks, it propels me into another classification in which I will earn more money and gain additional benefits."

(Look under "Resources" in the back of the book for locations of VA hospitals.)

RDH in a Long-Term Facility

Mary M. Masterson *discusses her career as a dental services coordinator in a private nursing home.*

I graduated in 1978 with a B.S. in Dental Hygiene. Since the school was in Oregon, I was now certified in local anesthesia, amalgam polishings and X-rays, as well as basic dental hygiene skills.

I believe that completion of a degree program opens up a broader range of employment opportunities because you then have a better understanding of public health education, research, the sciences, and patient education. I also believe that an administrator or director of a nursing home will be more inclined to hire someone with a degree because the hygienist will be more broadly qualified to direct a dental program.

I am currently employed in private practice three days a week and work two days a week in a Jewish nursing home. Before this position, I had left dental hygiene for a year because I saw very little room for future growth and development for myself. But during the period I was away I discovered I missed the personal contact I had with people, the independence that came with directing my skills and knowledge to the individual patient, and not being recognized as the professional I had trained for.

What To Do?

I became a dental claims auditor but didn't really enjoy it. I started looking for a dental hygiene position, having mixed emotions about returning. I feared that the feelings of boredom and disatisfaction would resurface once I was back.

One day a friend informed me of an advertisement in the paper for a dental hygienist in a nursing home. I was immediately intrigued with the uniqueness of this job possibility and sought an interview to see what expectations the nursing home had of a dental hygienist.

During the first interview, the interviewer explained that the job requirements were to set up and implement a dental program in the Home because some old donated dental equipment had recently been acquired. It was felt a dental hygienist could successfully develop and direct a dental program. Initially, the person would be needed for eight to 10 hours a month, but there was the possibility of increasing the hours as the program developed.

Out of the approximately 25 applicants interviewed, I was one of three asked to return. At the second interview, there were the expected questions of "Do you like working and being with elderly people?" "Do they bother you?" "Have you ever worked around sick or elderly people?" I responded that I had volunteered at a local hospital for four years as a junior auxiliary nurse and had helped care for my father for several years when he was bedridden. The one question that surprised me was "Do you feel you have a good sense of humor?" This was asked because things can become pretty chaotic and hectic, and if you can't laugh at yourself or the situation, you won't last very long in a nursing home! I said I felt I did, and explained how I had tried to get more information about the Home prior to my second interview.

What I Did

I had made up a letter stating my mother was in need of placement in a nursing home immediately. I wanted information regarding this facility because I had heard many positive comments on the quality of service and living conditions. I used a fictitious name and mailed the letter. The interviewers remembered the name because the letter was on file. The fictitious name I had used was the same name as one of their more "difficult" residents and they were hoping this potential resident wouldn't be as much of a problem! We all ended up laughing. I was offered the position and accepted it.

I felt the Home hired me because I had prior experience with the elderly, I had been out of school for a few years, I had graduated with a degree from a well-known institution, and I showed confidence in trying the new job. They said I would have full control in organizing the dental program since that was the reason they had hired me.

I felt the potential of the hours increasing with this job were very good and I could foresee a permanent dental program in the Home existing indefinitely. I believed the experience in the Home would be very interesting. In addition, I would be able to offer a service to a group of people in great need of dental care.

Starting the Program

Initially, there was no room for storing any equipment, no list of what needed to be attended to first, and no supplies. The donated equipment was stored at the Home. After discussion with the administrator and volunteer dentist, a budget was set aside to order basic supplies for doing oral assessments of the residents. The purpose of the assessments was to determine the needs of the Home, the dental status of the residents, and see what kind of response I would receive when introducing the dental program.

While I was performing the oral assessments, additional supplies were gradually ordered. The dental room was completed and the donated dental equipment installed.

Shortly after the used equipment was placed in the room, we received approval for new dental equipment to be donated by a local dental equipment manufacturer. After the initial request was sent to the dental manufacturer, I had to do several follow-up letters and phone calls before they gave us a commitment regarding the type of donation and delivery of the equipment to the Home. With the new equipment installed, we had a modern dental office ready for oral prophylaxes, exams and whatever else was required.

The dental room is equipped with a new dental chair that has arm rests that slide back and forth, rather than up and down. The mobile dental cart has a three-way syringe, two high-speed hookups, one low-speed hookup, a high-velocity vacuum system with a saliva ejector attachment, and a built-in ultrasonic unit with tips. There is an X-ray viewbox and a chemical sterilizer.

I established a dental charting system, a billing procedure, a recall system, a filing system, a written policy and procedures manual, and a written job description for a staff dentist and staff dental hygienist. When the original volunteer dentist stepped down from being dental director for the program, I had to approach someone else to fill this position. I was referred to the current dentist who visits the Home. He signed a contract with the Home and makes visits on a regular schedule to care for the residents. The time span for setting up the entire dental program was a sixteen-month period.

My Concerns

I had a few concerns when I began the job. I had no qualms about working with the residents or staff. My concerns were how to create a dental program that would run efficiently, blend in with the other departments, and be well received by staff, family members, residents, and my own professional colleagues. I had no previous experience in setting up a dental program/office and had to do a lot of consulting with several people, including the volunteer dentist who assisted in the initial planning of the program.

I think the issue of racial/cultural differences needs to be addressed, because I am experienced in this matter. I was born in Korea and was adopted and brought to the States at the age of three. Although I am Korean in heritage, I was raised an American. I was a bit nervous thinking that working in a Jewish nursing home might pose some problems. I thought that some of the residents, their families and friends, would have some kind of barrier about my being Korean, but I found this to be untrue. In fact, I found *my* ignorance of Jewish culture to be more of a problem.

For example, when I first began there, I was unaware of which foods were considered *Kosher* (a food approved by Rabbinical law). I had taken a small can of commercially-prepared chicken noodle soup into the main kitchen to be opened. This product had not been made from *Kosher* chicken. The dietician noticed me leaving the kitchen with an open can. She politely told me not to do this again and explained why. Anything *Kosher* is never to be used, mixed, or touched by a non-*Kosher* item. In this case, the can opener had touched the non-*Kosher* soup. What I am saying is it pays to study another group's culture!

Fitting In

I have found the dental program blending in well with the other departments at the Home. There is a team approach used with all the departments to determine the needs and method of treatment for a resident. For example, the physical therapist will ask me to evaluate a resident for loose dentures which might be the reason for an inadequate chewing process. Or the speech therapist will ask if patients can wear their dentures to improve speech. Also, I work with the dietician to change a diet texture if a patient will be without dentures for a period of time. If I am not able to make an evaluation, I arrange for the dentist to see the resident.

I feel the staff is very relieved to have someone who is adept in this area to field questions, complaints or concerns directed to them by residents and family members. This reduces the number of problems they must solve. The residents and family members like having someone available who will listen, explain, and follow through on a dental problem. To this point, I may have to call a dentist's office to see if a denture can be repaired the same day. I may have to deliver the denture to the office and arrange for the return to the resident if the resident is unable to make arrangements on their own. I do this to eliminate the time the resident will be without the prosthesis.

I help schedule appointments, obtain authorization from the physician before work is to be done, and communicate to family members what the resident will be having done. I find my greatest satisfaction to be when residents say that if I had not taken the time, they probably wouldn't have had it done because there was no one to take them to the office and the dentist was unable to come to the Home.

What I Like About the Job

My job encompasses many different roles at the nursing home that I normally would not be involved with in a private office. I work as a team member with the staff dentist. My title is dental services coordinator.

I act as a liaison for the dental program by working with the staff, residents, other health professionals, and dentists to get the work done. I have found this a very challenging and rewarding job. I have met many dentists here. This allows me to become familiar with others in the dental profession. I am able to interact with other health professionals and obtain knowledge through experiences with them. I have more responsibilities in the Home because the dentist, staff, residents and families rely on me to help with the decision-making.

I keep the dental and medical charts current with the resident's dental status, assist the dentist whenever possible, hold in-service meetings for the staff, and consult with the resident, family and staff.

I am allowed to do dental prophylaxes with the written authorization from the resident's attending dentist and physician. I have acquired a better understanding and acceptance of the elderly and am more comfortable around them. This has helped me accept and understand my own mother who is 72 years old.

I find that I would not want to return to private practice full time now that I have had a chance to experience working in a nursing home and know that I enjoy this kind of job.

What To Expect

You should know what compensation to expect when you work in a nursing home. You will probably be employed in two ways. First of all, the Home will hire you as a part-time employee. You will be considered an independent contractor and not receive any benefits. In the second way, the Home will contract a dentist to care for the residents. This dentist will pay your salary and any benefits. I am currently working as an independent contractor with the Home and submit my hours for payment. They do not provide any benefits for me.

I carry my own disability insurance because I am ineligible for worker's compensation. The Home will probably base your salary on a pay scale equivalent to their nurses. It might be advisable to accept their first salary offer, unless it is unreasonably low, and agree that a review and salary increase occur within three to six months. In my opinion, "low" ranges from $8.00 to $12.00 an hour. I would expect a salary increase of $2.00 to $5.00 an hour within the first year. The salary plateau you reach will depend on the financial status of the Home, how much education you have and continue to take, the amount of effort you put in the position, and how much responsibility you assume.

I feel the growth potential of dental hygiene careers in nursing homes is very good. The public is becoming more aware of the increasing population of people living longer and maintaining good health, dental health included. This segment of the population is demanding better health care in all areas of their living situations. The saturation of the dental profession in traditional settings is forcing dentists and dental hygienists to seek other potential areas of need. The nursing home population evidences an increasing need. When they see dental programs in nursing homes and volunteer dental in-services being implemented, administrators and their staff are more aware of and receptive to the introduction of a dental program in their facility.

Positions for dental hygienists in nursing homes will not be exactly the same as mine. Each home will be different in how they want the dental program set up and what their expectations of the dental hygienist will be.

Assessing Yourself

If you are interested in a job in this kind of setting, first ask yourself some questions:

• Do you enjoy working with elderly, and/or sick people? If you are unsure, volunteer at a local home or hospital.

• Will you be able to adapt to frequent patient schedule changes? For example, if a resident is not feeling well or has gone to the hospital, will you be able to fill that time with someone else or some other work?

• Does a person's title interfere with your needs or your ability to ask for something? If you must talk with the staff physician, will the fact that he is a doctor interfere with your effectiveness in talking with him? If so, you will need to overcome these feelings.

• Can you be relied on to adhere to your work schedule? This is an important factor because many people will be counting on you to help get the job done.

• Are you able to recognize when you need advice or assistance? The success of the program will depend on how well you meet the needs of the residents and follow through with the necessary procedures.

I would encourage anyone interested in this type of job to take the challenge and not let obstacles be a barrier to a rewarding and fulfilling career.

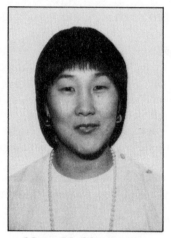

Mary M. Masterson

*[If you have any comments or questions, direct them to Mary M. Masterson, c/o **Career Directions Press**.]*

RDH in Education

RDH as an Educational Administrator

Sue Janusz *shows how re-entry into dental hygiene became her point of career change into dental hygiene education.*

I accepted my current position in educational administration 24 years after graduating from a dental hygiene program in the Midwest.

I then worked full time in a private dental office for three years. Though I enjoyed my work, I took a leave for a few years to raise my children. My husband was a graduate student during this period and we were moving around the country every one or two years. I decided to wait to return to private practice until we settled in one location.

Re-entry into Private Practice

My re-entry occurred after a six-year absence. Fortunately, there was a dental hygiene program in the community in which we settled and the director allowed me to use the facilities to update my skills. After a refresher period of several months, I passed the state board exam and received my license.

I returned to practice in a private dental office two days a week. I liked what I was doing and realized how much I had missed patient treatment and the social interaction which the profession offers. The additional income my salary provided was also welcomed.

My part-time employment continued for four years but was interrupted when my husband decided to take an academic sabbatical to the Northeast region of the United States. I regretted having to leave my position, but my employer assured me I could return to his practice as one of the dental hygienists in the group practice he was planning to form.

While living in the Northeast, I decided to return to college to take a few courses. I had been thinking about doing this for several years and wondered if I would be a successful student. At that point I had been out of school for 14 years.

After taking two courses at a small woman's college, I found I enjoyed the challenge of course work again and could succeed. In fact, the courses I took then and later seemed, in many cases, to be easier than my dental hygiene courses from years earlier!

Upon return to our community, I enrolled at the state university as a part-time student in the college of education. I also returned, on a part-time basis, to the same practice in which I had been promised a position on my return. I completed my bachelor's degree in education after one year.

Leaving Private Practice

I decided to leave private practice after my dentist/employer told me he wanted me to work full time. I told him I couldn't do that as I needed more of a challenge in my work routine.

About that same time I was offered, and accepted, a position as a part-time clinical instructor at the community college where I had done my refresher work a few years earlier. My dentist/employer then changed his mind and said that I could remain working at the office on a part-time basis. I had already decided to leave dental hygiene practice and devote my time to teaching students.

I believed that my years of practical experience and my maturity would be of educational value to dental hygiene students. I also realized, in our community of one hundred thousand people, I was only one of two RDHs over age thirty who had employment in private practice. It was my feeling that as I grew older, my skills would be less marketable in private dentistry. Now was the time to shift gears and focus my energies in a new career direction.

The Feelings That Change Can Bring

I felt a deep sense of loss when I left private practice even though I wasn't absolutely certain I was leaving permanently. Eight years of my professional life had been spent working closely with patients and dental staff. Leaving those interactions behind was quite difficult.

My feelings of loss quickly disappeared after I became a clinical instructor. I felt a keen sense of responsibility to the students whom I was teaching and to the institution in which I was employed. I wanted to be certain that I was teaching current information so when I was not instructing in the clinic, I audited didactic dental hygiene courses, read professional journals, and attended many continuing education courses.

51

Besides feeling responsible for teaching current information, I also felt required to be a good professional role model for students. I knew the effect role modeling had on young children but was still too new to realize fully the impact a teacher can have on adult students until I had taught for a few weeks. Hearing students speak to their patients in the same tone of voice or with the same vocabulary as I had used with them was often quite revealing!

I had been admitted to graduate school during this period. A full-time faculty position in the dental hygiene program at the college also opened up. An instructor was needed to teach clinic seminar courses and the course in oral and dental anatomy. I knew that a good deal of time and effort would be necessary to be a good classroom teacher and I was willing to devote myself to the work involved.

I had enjoyed the classroom student teaching which I had done a few years earlier (some of which was in oral and dental anatomy) and believed I had the necessary qualifications and attitude to do the job. I applied for the position. After several interviews with college administrators, I was offered and accepted the position.

I didn't know how many other applicants there were for this job. I believed that my degree in education, my years of private practice, and my personal commitment to my students, my colleagues and the college, were probably the deciding factors in getting the offer.

I decided to withdraw from graduate school after one semester so that I could devote all my time to my new teaching position. I continued to teach full time, and, after one year, returned to graduate school. After four years I completed my master's degree in education.

Moving Up

My graduate advisor often asked me if I planned to become a dental hygiene program coordinator in the future. I always replied that I was content with didactic and laboratory clinical instruction. However, my attitude towards administrative responsibilities changed when the coordinator's position in the program in which I teach became available.

I accepted the job as co-coordinator of the program after many discussions, meetings and interviews with the administrators. I decided I was ready to change my position and accept new challenges.

Then in January 1987 my responsibilities changed again. I am now the sole coordinator of the dental hygiene program.

Requirements for an administrative position in our college include a master's degree, teaching experience, and the ability to perform administrative tasks. Salaries range from $25,000-$30,000, depending on one's background.

Our college has an excellent benefits package including membership in a state retirement system, medical and dental insurance, cost-of-living salary increases, and regular academic salary increases. Academic breaks, though often "working breaks," allow some time for refreshing one's self.

What the Job Entails

The work at times seems endless. After one task is completed, several others appear which often require immediate attention.

Much of the responsibility in this position involves attending college division meetings, conducting staff meetings, developing program policy, working with the clinic supervisor on clinical operations, evaluating faculty, advising and teaching.

Time must also be devoted to tasks involving national, state and local professional organizations, and the community and surrounding district in which our college exists.

All of these duties make the job varied, challenging and fast-paced. The work is never boring or at a standstill. I enjoy the multiple aspects. I particularly enjoy the innovation I am able to bring to the program and the support and assistance I am able to give the faculty and students to encourage their personal and professional development.

My greatest reward comes from the realization that the entire profession and society benefits from our collective efforts.

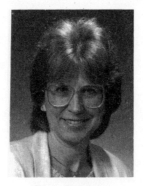

Sue Janusz

53

RDH as an Educational Consultant

Shawn O'Neill-Hoffman brings the latest research to practicing dental professionals through her position as educational consultant in the dental industry.

Hygienists are always asking me how I became involved as an educator with a dental company. I must admit my career has been the result of being in the right place at the right time and with the right credentials. I have many hygienists to thank as, when they became pregnant while working at their respective jobs, opportunities became available for me. These ranged from clinical hygiene positions to my current role as an educational consultant with *Teledyne Water Pik*, a company devoted to improving oral health through the marketing of unique, innovative products.

I work with three very talented hygienists; together we make up the professional educational division of *Teledyne Water Pik*. We attend all major dental meetings as well as present continuing education seminars for dentists and hygienists. Our goal is to keep the profession abreast of the most recent research regarding periodontal disease.

The job entails extensive travel nationwide with all expenses paid. We work on a contractual, part-time basis with salaries ranging between $115 to $150 per day, based on years of experience with the company.

Each of our backgrounds varies although basic requirements include a bachelor's degree, at least two years of private practice experience, and public speaking before large groups.

By combining our professional consulting with clinical practice, we are aware of the trends occurring in dentistry and how these changes may impact the marketplace. We provide a link between the dental profession and a dentally-related company.

Clinical Practice or More School?

When I graduated from dental hygiene school in 1977, I really had no idea what I was getting myself into. I've always loved the school environment and I wasn't sure if I was ready to enter the working world.

My first experience as a dental hygienist was in a hectic general practice in a metropolitan area in the Midwest. I can see how hygienists could burn out as I lasted only one summer before returning to school.

My next stop was the University of Missouri at Kansas City where I worked on my Bachelor of Science Degree in Dental Hygiene. At this point, teaching hygiene appeared to be an excellent alternative to clinical practice. I also had thoughts of going on to dental school one day, so I enrolled in predental courses.

Due to financial necessity, I joined a periodontal office after I graduated from UMKC. As much as I enjoyed periodontics, I was still seeking alternatives. A year and a half later, I packed up my bags again and moved to Boston to work on a master's degree in dental public health. I left behind my boyfriend (now husband) who was very understanding and supportive.

When I finished the program at Boston University, I moved back home to my parents. I wanted to secure a position before moving to Denver where my husband had been transferred. I worked part-time as a clinical dental hygiene instructor at a local college and filled in as a hygienist for a general dentist.

In order to better market myself, I enrolled in a job placement course which prepared me for interviews and job negotiations. I had two résumés professionally prepared—one geared with a teaching position in mind and one tailored for a sales position.

At that time, public health opportunities in large cities were not available. My father was instrumental in getting me to consider areas of sales or marketing.

Getting Interviews

On my first trip to Denver, I had arranged to meet with the director of professional services at *Teledyne Water Pik.* We discussed my future goals and impending relocation to Colorado. In 1980, *Teledyne Water Pik* was one of the few companies hiring hygienists specifically for their skills, both clinical and academic. Unfortunately, the position in Denver was taken, but the director said she would keep my résumé on file. This one informal interview was very positive even though I didn't leave with a job offer. There is a nice, close network of people in the dental industry and I left Fort Collins with a list of potential contacts, as well as a new reference.

I also met with the director of the dental hygiene program at the University of Colorado. Although there were no openings at the school, I was furnished with another list of contacts. Securing a job in Denver while living on the East Coast was difficult, to say the least, so I finally made the big move in the latter part of that year.

I decided to continue pursuing other areas while practicing hygiene. I was hired by a periodontist to substitute for his pregnant hygienist. This led to a mutually convenient work schedule.

I had finally found a dentist with whom I felt comfortable working and one who respected me. This was the perfect outlet to apply my clinical skills and periodontal knowledge.

To supplement my clinical abilities, I became involved preparing educational modules for dental assisting students. One of my contacts finally paid off! I worked at home in my free time and was paid hourly. I really enjoyed the diversity.

Within a few months, I had met with most of my contacts. I also attended the Denver Midwinter Meeting to introduce myself to the dental industry. Most companies were impressed by my background, but reluctant to hire anyone without sales experience. To this day, I don't know where one is supposed to get sales experience if no one is willing to give you a chance! *Teledyne Water Pik's* Professional Services Department was looking more attractive with each interview.

Although I was quite happy with the periodontal office, I needed some other type of fulfillment. I wanted to unleash all my energy and background as an educator and hygienist with an advanced degree.

The following summer changed all that. I had interviewed for the position of director of the dental assisting program at a local college and was, at the same time, contacted by *Teledyne Water Pik.* They told me that the Denver hygienist was pregnant and they were interested in having me replace her.

After eight months of interviews, I had been offered two positions in one day! I was interested in both but it finally boiled down to the exposure, visibility, and professional and personal growth offered by *Teledyne Water Pik.* Besides, my first dental meeting would be in San Francisco. Who could refuse!

Four years later, the travel is much less appealing. Many times I only see an airport, hotel, and lecture or exhibit hall. The real gratification comes from presenting a seminar to groups of dentists and hygienists, thereby increasing their level of awareness and interest. We have lectured to graduate students and many times this has helped to spur or stimulate research at the university level. Another source of gratification for me.

The preparation for our seminars cannot be done the night before; the knowledge is cumulative. As a hygienist in private practice, I don't believe I read half as many volumes of clinical research in one year compared to what I'm now reviewing monthly. As motivators and educators, each consultant has to be on top of the latest findings and be able to communicate the clinical research to the practicing professional.

Because of our high visibility, many of us have been approached by other dental companies who are interested in developing programs such as ours. Although their salaries and fringe benefits may be attractive, our core group has remained fairly stable. This is an exciting time for products such as ours and we thrive on the challenge of presenting new information, as well as information that has been misunderstood in the past and, therefore, ignored or not utilized fully in private practice. We realize how busy hygienists and dentists are with their daily schedules. We hope we are providing a valuable service in our dissemination of the literature.

Approaching Companies

My advice to RDHs contemplating similar work would be to:

(1) create your own position;

(2) demonstrate the need and show your talents to companies;

(3) get in there and make personal contacts;

(4) don't forego your clinical experience; it is a necessary prerequisite.

Presently, I reside in Oregon. I am busy scheduling my spring lectures and updating my slide presentation. I continue to practice with the periodontal group in Denver whenever I'm in town.

I'm definitely in a unique position and have come to realize how important clinical hygiene really is. I'm able to apply the knowledge I've gained through my position with *Teledyne Water Pik* and feel more aware that I know what's going on with my patients.

Because of my dual role, I believe I've become a more effective clinician and my level of patient care has greatly improved. In short, I enjoy hygiene even more because I can see the relevance of research to my patient's progress. I like being a dental hygienist.

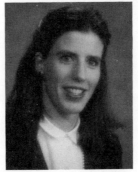

Shawn O'Neill-Hoffman

Margarita Ayala *tells us of reaching her career goals through her role as educator of dental hygiene students.*

I received an Associate of Applied Science degree in Dental Hygiene 21 years ago from the State University of New York at Farmingdale. Graduation day, as I recall, was one full of excitement and a great sense of accomplishment. I am number six out of twelve children and was the first to attend and graduate from college. The fact that I was the college valedictorian made my parents, family and college sponsor extremely proud, and gave *me* great satisfaction in knowing that the countless hours devoted to studying were being recognized and rewarded.

At this point, I felt I needed a rest before embarking on my job-hunting mission. I used the summer period to work as a waitress in a camp for mentally handicapped children.

When I returned at the end of August, I started looking at want ads for a clinic or hospital dental hygiene position. I imagined I would feel comfortable working in a clinic/hospital environment, since my experiences with dental treatment had been in that type of arrangement. I was also considering the fringe benefits which are part of most municipal jobs.

Getting a Job

Just prior to my going on interviews, I was offered a full-time dental hygiene teaching position as a technical assistant at the college from which I had just graduated. The starting salary at that time was about $4800 per year. (Remember, this is over twenty years ago!) Now this offer put me in a quandry as to how I would proceed with my life.

On one hand, I was ready to get a position where I would be using my newly-acquired skills in providing oral health services to the public. On the other hand, teaching was a profession I had never considered.

I was always a very quiet and introverted person and the idea of standing in front of a group and lecturing terrified me. I was assured the position involved mostly clinical and laboratory classes where I would be working in a one-to-one or small-group situation. I accepted the position because it offered a big challenge to my basic personality and I wanted to find out if I would overcome my fear and, perhaps, even *like* my new role and responsibilities.

What I Learned

After one year of full-time teaching, my entire outlook on it changed! From trembling in front of students the first few weeks, I acquired more self-confidence with each passing day that I survived the ordeal. When I saw that students were human beings like myself, with fears and anxieties of their own, I began to relax and put my fears aside to concentrate on imparting my knowledge to them. By the end of the year, I felt very comfortable in my new position and was actually enjoying my new role.

The Next Step

In order to maintain and advance in my position, I began to think about furthering my education and obtaining an advanced degree. I matriculated on a part-time basis at a major New York university and took some courses during the summer and evenings of the following academic year. Marriage, children and family obligations caused me to interrupt my pursuit of a bachelor's degree.

After seven years as a technical assistant, I resigned from the position to raise my family. Ten years after I received my associate degree, while my children were still small, I returned to college on a full-time basis to earn my bachelor's and master's degree in dental hygiene education. I had acquired a love for teaching! To increase my chances of obtaining a position in education again, I knew I would have to make sacrifices (financially, physically and mentally) to get my degrees. As you can imagine, it was a difficult task to attend school with two small children. Without my husband's full support, I could not have attained my goals.

Competing for Jobs

Upon completion of my master's degree in 1979, I applied to several dental hygiene programs in the New York City area for a teaching position. I was hired as a full-time assistant professor at the same school I had attended and previously taught in. The job requirements were that the applicant have a master's degree, two years of dental hygiene teaching experience and two years of clinical practice. The salary range was between $16,000 and $18,000 per year. Fringe benefits included pension plan, dental and medical benefits, prescription drug plan, vision plan, paid sick and vacation time. (Faculty have a ten-month obligation which frees the summer months for personal enjoyment.)

The applicant pool was quite competitive since not many full-time teaching positions become available in this area. I was picked for the position because I more than met all the qualifications, plus I had seven years of teaching experience at Farmingdale. I also had a recent degree in dental hygiene education which is considered the terminal degree in dental hygiene. The fact that I was a minority, I feel, was another factor.

My responsibilities include teaching and coordinating the radiology lecture and laboratory course, as well as instructing in the preclinical and clinical courses. I have also been the SADHA co-advisor for the past five years.

Moving Upward

The chances for advancement in this position are good. I received tenure this past year and was promoted to associate professor. My salary has about doubled in eight years.

This position fills my needs in various respects. Since I have a family, it allows me to spend a great deal of time with them. The other aspect is the satisfaction I obtain from teaching. I find it challenging, exciting and rewarding to see students grow and progress from day one until graduation. I enjoy working with people and I try to treat each student as an individual with different capabilities. My role as a teacher is to help students achieve their full potential and reach their goals.

In addition to my full-time position, I have been an adjunct assistant professor of dental hygiene at Hostos Community College in New York City for the past eight years. At this college, my responsibilities include instructing in the first-year preclinic and clinic sequence, and for the past three years I have coordinated and taught the radiology lecture and laboratory course.

Staying on Top

During summer months and on some weekends, I occasionally work in private practice. I feel this is a must for every dental hygiene educator to help us keep abreast of the latest developments and stay in tune with reality. I think this experience makes me a more well-rounded educator and better role model for students.

I find dental hygiene to be an exciting career and profession. It has allowed me mobility and flexibility to meet my personal needs. I was able to climb the career ladder into the specialized area of education.

At the same time, it has given me the flexibility I need to maintain a home with two teenage boys and an eight-month old baby girl, in addition to holding a full and part-time teaching position.

I have found through my years of experience that *determination* assisted me in overcoming the many obstacles that seemed to hinder the achievement of my goals. I am very happy with my choices.

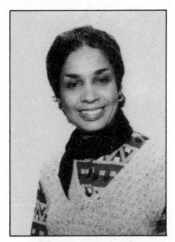

Margarita Ayala

External Degrees

External Degree Programs—A Boon for the Self-Disciplined

Acquiring a bachelor's or master's degree through an accredited external degree program can be a time- and cost-efficient way for motivated RDHs to meet their educational objectives.

Such a degree comes from your participation in the awarding institution's program and is based on their evaluation of your accredited and non-accredited coursework. An external degree program is highly individualized in its concept and its approach to your learning experiences.

The main advantages to pursuing such a course of education is that

- Little or no time is spent in the classroom.
- Credit for non-traditional learning can be awarded (continuing education and life experiences, for example.)
- There are flexible entrance requirements.
- Learning is at your own pace.
- You can still work full time.

This is *not* a route for someone who lacks self-discipline or self-motivation. You have to be able to work independently and be a full partner in your learning experience.

Here are some degree-awarding, fully-accredited programs (by the parent university and regional accrediting agencies) that have been checked for credibility.

School	Degree	Contact
St. Joseph's College—External Degree Services Roanoke, VA	Bachelor's degree in Health Care Admin. and Business Administration	800/336-9622
Vermont college of Norwich Univ. Montpelier, VT	Bachelor's degrees in Liberal Arts, Public Health Admin., Bus. Admin., Counseling (Master's program available.)	800/332-1987 (In Vt. call 800/553-3326)
Syracuse Univ.-Independent Study Degree Programs Syracuse, NY	Bachelor's degrees in Bus. Admin., Liberal Studies (MBA also available)	315/423-3284
Continuing and Int'l. Education Antioch Univ. Yellow Springs, OH	Master's degree curriculum tailored to educational and career goals	513/767-1031 -2661

When you call, *qualify* the school by asking:
— What are the requirements for enrollment?
— Do I receive credit for previous studies/life experience?
— Is there a deadline for completion?
— Is there any residency requirement?
— What are the fees involved? How must they be paid?
— How do I communicate with my instructors?

Ask that a catalog of programs and available literature be sent to you so that you can see if what's being offered meets your needs.

(Look under "Resources" in the back of the book for names and addresses of post-certificate educational programs. For a complete listing, write to the American Assoc. of Dental Schools, 1625 Mass. Ave., N.W., Wash., D.C. 20036)

Be Sure You Need A Degree

Any degree, graduate or otherwise, is only of value *if you have a purpose in getting one.* Degrees for their own sake, while they can't hurt, do not focus your thinking *to a specific objective.*

First comes targeting your goal. Then lay out your plans for reaching it. Formal education may be a necessary credential for what you want to do (it is for practicing dental hygiene!), or it may not. *But it should not be an end in itself* for someone exploring career options.

For example, if you want to go into dental research, a master's degree will probably be a necessity but *there is no guarantee it will get you a job.* How much wiser to investigate research centers in schools and hospitals, talking to people who are doing that type of work. Find out exactly what it is you have to do to get your foot in the door. You may find that you can do some work part-time or volunteering. This experience will point you to the degree program most suitable for the direction you want to take. Or, you may find that research is not what you expected and decide it's not for you. You now have the knowledge to set your direction elsewhere.

Once you've determined what you are interested in doing, find out if jobs exist in your area by contacting organizations and facilities in which those activities are performed. Ask what the necessary qualifications are for filling such a position. You will then have a more realistic idea of what you need to know to qualify yourself. Now "fill in the holes". Keep in mind that nowhere is it written you will automatically earn more money if you have more schooling. Or even guarantee you the assurance of a job.

65

Knowing What You Want—First

According to Richard Nelson Bolles, the guru of career counselors, there are five reasons why most people want to go back to school.

(1) They want to acquire more knowledge about a subject for intellectual rather than vocational reasons;

(2) they want to pick up additional, marketable skills to help them advance in their present field;

(3) they want to acquire the requisite skills to change fields;

(4) they want to stretch their mental capacity by undertaking an intellectually rigorous course of study;

(5) they want relief from the world of work (otherwise known as "the perpetual student syndrome".

Which reason, or combination of reasons, applies to you?

Many times RDHs become professional students. That is to say, they take courses endlessly in the hope of finding a clue as to which career direction they should pursue. The reason why the task is endless is that they are going about it in reverse. Additional schooling is the means to the objective. If there is no objective, the means continue in a non-directed fashion and never really assume a shape.

Clarify your thinking as to what you want. Then find out if more schooling will bring you to fulfilling that dream. If you know what you want *before* you go after it, you will not be disappointed in the outcome.

RDH As Consultant

RDH as Consultant for Patients and Practices

J. Patricia Thatcher *offers a most unusual service in her counseling/consulting practice on patient management.*

What I Believe

I am an adventurer at heart. By this I mean that I perceive life as a series of challenges which often require courage, intelligence, fortitude, an intuitive awareness and a keen sense of excitement. My choice to become a counselor and consultant is directly related to this spirit. I believe people can meet their fears and anxieties with courage because the energy produced can then be used to aid growth in a more productive, satisfying way. As a dental hygienist, I often experience people who are in an anxious and fearful state. My desire to help these people led me to seek the knowledge and techniques useful in relieving these responses. This, in turn, led me to teach other health professionals ways in which to relieve anxiety both in their patients as well as in themselves.

I actually made the decision to become a full-time counselor/consultant in 1983. I was taking an advanced class in Eriksonian Hypnosis. At some moment during that class it became clear to me that I wanted to use the knowledge and techniques available to me to help people overcome their fears. Yet, there were many events, both personal and professional, which led me to decide on this course of action.

How It All Began

In 1969, when I graduated from dental hygiene school, I was 21 years old. Like many new graduates, I thought little about dental hygiene as a *career*. It was a way to help people in need and to make a little money while I decided what to do with the rest of my life.

Finally, after ten years as a dental hygienist, it occured to me that I *had* a career. Those ten years were exciting and enriching ones in many respects. In other respects, they were disappointing and always left me with a hunger for more.

It seems to me that I played a game which I have termed "Career-go-round." It is a little like merry-go-round blown up to life-size proportions and it goes something like this:

Upon graduation from hygiene school I worked in a private practice—got bored—joined a medical/dental relief organization, worked in Appalachia for 15 months—burned out—moved to Boston and worked in public health in an urban health center—again burned out—moved back into private practice—got bored, and then worked in a toothpaste research project.

By the age of 27 I had a series of jobs (some more interesting than others), all of which gave me immeasurable experience—and all of which always left me wanting something I could not express. I seemed to be going round and round trying to catch the ring, but just missing it.

The one thread which connected all these different roles was my ability to work with individuals in a way that changed their lives. Each person I saw left with a new motivation and a sense of importance. It was this individual work with patients which kept me in dental hygiene. I continually sought personal growth experiences and courses to help me be a better motivator and teacher as well as continued to learn clinical techniques useful in treating periodontal and caries problems. Looking back now, it seems to me I was trying to incorporate my need for adventure and excitement into my professional work schedule. I did not always succeed.

Developing New Skills

I became more aware of my adventurous spirit when I returned to school for my bachelor's degree in health education. This was the change I needed to seek new directions; it triggered a series of events which continues to influence my life.

I worked hard in school, but also tested my physical capabilities by scuba diving, completing *Outward Bound,* sky diving and backpacking in the hills of Vermont. We often set our limits too low and I learned that most people are capable of accomplishing much more than they realize they can. I had to face my own fears and found that I came out on the other side a stronger and more enriched person. I now *knew* I could do those things I always wanted to do but was too afraid to try.

After completing my studies, I decided to take a sojourn around this country, giving myself a year. After nine months, however, as I was camping in the Colorado Mountains, my mother died. I returned to Boston, distraught and nearly penniless, but rich in the warmth, love and support of good friends. Because of my poor finances and a need to be productive, it was very easy to fall back into my old routine.

Luckily, I came in contact with a prosthodontist who wanted a hygienist to help him build a high-quality, patient-oriented practice. I accepted this position using all my expertise and knowledge to ensure continual growth. Because of the prosthetic specialty, we often saw people who needed serious, complicated and expensive treatment. Patients frequently exhibited fear and anxiety about this treatment, while others had a history of dental phobia which prevented them from seeking care in the early stages of dental disease. I saw I needed better skills to relieve this anxiety and to help people through the many months of treatment and so began a nine-month training in the humanistic therapies where I learned information and techniques useful in relieving anxiety.

Other skills were also useful in motivating people to care for their health. I used every available resource including referring patients to therapists when it seemed necessary. At the same time I continued to study those psychologies pertinent to my needs, especially those areas relating to the work of Milton Erikson and medical hypnosis.

As the practice grew and the recall system began to function properly, I saw more and more routine patients. There were always a few problem and hard-to-motivate people, but once I spent some time with them relieving their anxieties, they needed only maintenance care. That old haunt, boredom, began to set in as there were less challenges in my daily schedule. I was no longer penniless; I decided to take a trip!

I asked for a six-month leave of absence in order to tour the world. One of my goals was to locate and write about dental hygienists in other countries. This gave me an excellent avenue through which to meet new people and to experience a part of the culture not accessible to the normal tourist. A productive benefit was an article I wrote for *RDH* magazine (Nov./Dec. 1982) describing my experiences.

When I returned to the States six months later, I found that both I and the practice had changed. The practice had grown, incorporated, and expanded to new office space. But my role did not grow with it. I was now expected to keep to an inflexible, more traditional job description for dental hygiene. I became more dissatisfied as each week passed.

It seemed the only professional excitement I had were the times I was able to use my skills in helping phobic, anxious, and hard-to-motivate patients. I continued to study the humanistic therapies and taught a course for dental hygienists on the use of these skills in their own lives. It was very successful and I loved teaching peer professionals.

While I knew it was time for a major career change, I did not know in which direction to turn. There were few resources available to me and fewer role models. I did not want to get back into playing "Career-go-round" again, so I bided my time while deciding what to do.

I started drawing up lists stating my requirements for satisfaction. These included:

> I wanted to be more in charge of my daily schedule.
>
> I wanted to be my own boss.
>
> I wanted to use my intelligence and creativity.
>
> I wanted to use my psychological skills and training on a more ongoing basis.
>
> I wanted to help people grow by relieving their dental anxiety as well as other fears and phobias.
>
> I wanted to make more money.
>
> I wanted to use my adventurous spirit in my daily work plan and incorporate my love for backpacking into my professional life.
>
> I wanted to stop doing daily, routine clinical dental hygiene.
>
> I wanted to empower other hygienists to be more successful with their patients and their lives.

As much as I enjoyed working with individual patients, office policies in most practices fail to give hygienists the motivation and flexibility necessary to continue their personal and professional growth. I considered many other options including retraining in a different field. However, I had a tremendous amount of time and experience invested in this career. What I needed was an avenue to expand upon this experience.

Opening the Door

I realized there was a market for my services since there are over 19 million people who do not go to the dentist because of fear, and millions more who go but with trembling feet. Other statistics show that close to 30 million people suffer from irrational fears and phobias but only about two percent are treated.

I asked myself, "Why can't I begin a private counseling practice where I can successfully help people find relief from their fears and phobias?" The only thing which stopped me was my own lack of confidence, so I began to build self-confidence by focusing on the successes I had with my patients and my continuing education classes.

I also spoke with the teachers with whom I had trained. These were people I respected and they gave me much encouragement. It seemed that what I risked most was financial ruin, and, while this is still a consideration, no one succeeds without risk. I set out on a new adventure.

71

The first thing I did was attend a workshop for women beginning a consulting business. I then designed a counseling/consulting practice the primary goal of which is to relieve anxieties and fears which prevent people from functioning in some aspect of their lives. The main focus is on—but not limited to—treating dental anxiety as well as offering referral services for those who need gentle, competent dental care.

As a corollary to this, my backpacking partner and I decided to lead small groups on beginner and intermediate backpacking trips. Both she and I have found this to be an excellent opportunity to help people (especially women) gain new confidence in themselves. This, in turn, has positive spinoff effects in many other areas of their lives.

I gave my notice at the office, agreeing to work one day a week to treat patients who have phobic problems. I negotiated as an independent contractor at a higher pay scale. This gave me the assurance of ongoing financial support while giving the practice the continued marketing value provided by my services.

I had business cards and stationery printed, sent opening announcements, began to schedule more continuing education classes, wrote several articles, and gave small talks to professionals about my services.

On the advice of my sister, I contacted a specialist in the Small Business Development Corporation (a subsidiary of the Small Business Administration) offering free business counseling. The woman working with me has given me invaluable advice on developing a business plan and marketing my services.

Setting Goals

Initially, I gave myself one year to be successful. I have since extended that goal to three to five years. It takes time, patience and much hard work to build a counseling practice. The techniques I use are very effective and take a relatively short amount of time. As a result, I need a constant turnover of clients. Successful people refer others; a slow but sure process of continual growth.

At first, the financial benefits are poor, but the potential monetary rewards far exceed the pay scale for clinical dental hygiene, and there are many tax benefits available for someone in business. My level of personal satisfaction has increased greatly. At last I have a profession which allows me to incorporate my skills, creativity and sense of adventure into my life as a whole.

Some of the other fringe benefits include flexibility in scheduling. I can now schedule my daily routine according to my needs as well as schedule appropriate time for client needs with no outside inter-ference. I also have the opportunity to effect positive change in other peoples' lives (health professionals included), as well as the general public seeking relief from their anxieties.

Any good business plan includes a future vision. Mine is to return to school for a graduate degree in psychiatric social work. My inten-tions are to help people get in touch with and use those inner resources which will help them to be healthier human beings. I hope to use coun-seling services, continuing education and outdoor adventures to lead people to seek their potentials.

Anaïs Nin once said that the world at large will only become a bet-ter place to live when each individual finds personal freedom and satis-faction. I hope to help some of those people, including myself, do just that.

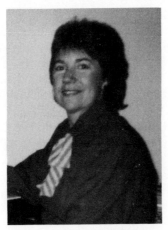

J. Patricia Thatcher

*(Interested readers can contact J. Patricia Thatcher through **Career Directions for Dental Hygienists**.)*

RDH as Consultant for Practices and Agencies

Phebe Blitz *outlines her move to incorporate her administrative skills into a practice management consultancy.*

The Challenge of Change

My career has been a growth process evolving over a long period of time in response to changes within myself and changes within my environment. At times this process has been very frustrating, especially when I found myself in a new area of the country and seemingly had to start over again. Most of the time, however, the process has been very rewarding.

At present, I am setting up a personal corporation to help me define, develop and administer my professional endeavors and goals. One of my undertakings includes managing a dental hygiene department in a private dental office. The administration of this department involves planning the system of care, designing appropriate records, maintaining inventory control, developing and evaluating personnel, overseeing financial planning, and providing direct patient services.

Other dimensions of my venture offer consultation and educational services to health care agencies and providers on practice management, emergency care, communications and marketing. I plan, market, arrange facilities, conduct programs, and evaluate the services for which I have contracted. For all of this, the ability to organize and communicate are crucial.

My interest in management, particularly administrative tasks, developed gradually. When I graduated from dental hygiene school, I worked for a year and a half and then gratefully retired to become a suburban housewife and mother. Always thankful to have the security of dental hygiene tucked safely away.

Re-entry into Education

After seven years of managing children and a household, I decided to re-enter the workforce. I took a hard look at myself, evaluating my capabilities and my career interests. After considering many other fields, I found that dental hygiene had a lot to offer. I decided to re-enter the profession and head for a career in dental hygiene education. I had taught swimming for years and *knew* I liked teaching.

I now lived in another state and had never felt it necessary to get a license to practice. So nine years after graduating I took the licensing examination. To my amazement I passed the first time! In order to become current, I looked for a job one day a week and called the closest dental hygiene school to inquire about continuing education courses. I made an appointment to discuss my career (where and how to start) with the director of a dental hygiene program at a major dental school nearby.

From that person, I received lots of support and encouragement as well as specific information on available teaching positions and educational opportunities. I enrolled in a master's program to get a degree in dental hygiene education and administration. During the next three years I attended classes, worked in private practice, and taught in a clinic part time. These three activities had a synergistic effect on each other and offered me maximum benefits.

Combining Administration into the Job

After completing my degree, I took a position which combined education and administration. I was coordinating the second-year clinical course in a dental hygiene school. Although I saw the position as one in education, I had ample opportunity to develop my administrative skills.

The director of the program served as an excellent role model in managing people and organizing work. She also provided a lot of support for personal and professional development. When an opening for a director of dental hygiene became available, I decided to apply. I didn't think I wanted the position, but I did want the experience of the interview process. (The process consisted of several group and several individual interviews.) With the information gained during the process, I decided to take the position.

The job consisted of leading eleven faculty and three staff to implement two curriculums. It included management of student admissions and records, financial control, clinical maintenance and operation, curriculum development and evaluation.

A lot of time in a position such as this is spent communicating and negotiating with faculty and administrators in the dental school and throughout the university.

A significant amount of time also is required for planning and organizing, but a typical day seldom goes as planned. So the key to success is often flexibility. A successful administrator must be able to assess, prioritize, delegate and follow-up—many of the same skills it takes to manage a household and organize children.

75

Enter Managing

It was in this position that I developed my managerial skills. I could see and feel first-hand the effectiveness of my capabilities. The expression "experience is a dear teacher" was certainly true in this situation. I learned very quickly from my mistakes. I also had opportunities to attend several workshops on administration during that time.

After three years in this position I was forced to evaluate my career. I had, in fact, developed my skills and enjoyed the work tremendously. I had accomplished all my original goals in three years. However, some personal changes had occurred in my life.

I was divorced and therefore had to look at long-term financial security. Although my position was secure, it did not pay me enough to live comfortably in my present environment, a suburb of New York City. I could be assured of automatic raises negotiated by the union but they barely kept up with the ever-rising cost of living. When I looked at career mobility from that position, I didn't see any. The next step up would have been as an assistant dean, and that, in this institution, would have been an impossible move for a dental hygienist. Because the dental school was somewhat removed from the rest of the university and the workloads were greater, there was little opportunity to move upward in other areas.

I did not consider the workload and pressure healthy for a long-term situation. I decided to make a change.

Reasons for Change

At this point in my life I was confident in my professional skills and needed to explore and develop myself as a person. So the decisions I made were more for personal reasons than professional ones. I chose to move to San Francisco. It offered a big-city atmosphere with a healthy life style. Dental hygiene was progressive there and the salary was better than on the East Coast.

I spent one and one-half years in San Francisco, thoroughly enjoying the city and getting to know myself. I used my network of professional contacts to locate jobs in private practice. I had to rebuild my career in the new location. I found it somewhat frustrating to have to prove myself again. Although I had help from my network, I found many people very threatened by my arrival. I wanted to use my new organizational and communication skills in a productive and progressive way immediately, but found it took time in a new location to develop the credibility I had taken for granted in New York. As I was ready to leave California, I could see I was beginning to develop credibility again.

Another big personal decision, to try marriage for the second time, necessitated another geographic move. This time, to Arizona.

I expected a difficult move professionally. I again used my network of association colleagues, but this time, I found an open reception.

Through the association placement service I found a job in private practice part-time to support myself while getting settled in a new area. The dentist/employer recognized my organizational and communication skills and encouraged me to use them in the practice. What started out to be one day a week cleaning teeth has turned into three days a week managing and developing the dental hygiene department.

Enter Consulting

As I worked to broaden the department, it occurred to me that other offices could use help in building their practices. My employer, in fact, suggested we might be able to help a friend of his. With that lead, a colleague and I developed a program to help other offices expand their practices.

Our program consists of several offerings:
(1) Group process sessions to determine the philosophy and goals for the office.
(2) Consultation on specific issues raised by the office.
(3) Work sessions to demonstrate and develop patient care strategies.
(4) Evaluation of treatments and identification of profit centers.
(5) Identification and development of individual personnel strengths.

We have only used word of mouth to market our services so far. We will use more aggressive marketing strategies as the program is tested and modified.

This is one example of ways to use education, experience, and skills to provide a service to fulfill a need. It comes from working hard in one direction while keeping an open mind to see opportunities or to *make* them, after seeing other problem areas.

Building on a Foundation

In working with many hygienists and offices in different areas of the country, I have been able to identify common problems and discover solutions from one area that can be applied to another. With my experience in education, I have developed several seminars and continuing education courses to share these solutions for common

77

problems. These seminars also serve to market the consulting services and build contacts in my new location.

With all these activities going on (but no one as much as I would like), it is easy to feel frustrated and fragmented. Sometimes I feel as if there are no opportunities in this part of the country. Sometimes I feel as if I don't have time to go after and develop any one pursuit. There are also financial realities. I just cannot afford to go without an income while I develop something that may pay off in the future. I need to be able to put food on the table regularly.

These feelings, as well as my need for future security, led me to investigate forming a corporation. Although I found that legal incorporation would have no financial advantages unless my income was approximately $60,000, I found that looking at my professional activities as a corporation helped me to organize them. It helped me see relationships between previously unrelated activities. It helped me see successes instead of being overwhelmed by how much still remained to be done.

Now I can look at the overall picture and make decisions that have a positive effect on all the areas. It has helped me plan, market, organize, control and evaluate my undertakings.

At this point, I earn the same as in private practice. By forming a corporation, I hope to increase my income and provide benefits and security for myself for the future. I will then have the flexibility to be involved in a variety of projects without losing my security.

My career—like my life—has not been a straight, level path. There have been changes in direction, and many hills and valleys. Likewise, there was not one decision that changed my career. Rather, it has evolved over a period of time as a result of personal frustration and environmental changes.

How I See Myself

There are two parts of my personality that have been responsible for the changes. One is a part of me that is very idealistic and likes to get things done in the most effective and efficient manner possible. I call that part of me *The Perfectionist. The Perfectionist* is seldom satisfied with reality and is usually frustrated. This frustration has been a tremendous motivator to make changes.

The other part of me is *The Challenger.* I enjoy trying new things; I always learn about myself. Many times it has been difficult to leave the security of *what is* to take a risk for *what might be.* But, because I enjoy a challenge, I have been able to take risks—and grow!

78

During my career development, I have practiced dental hygiene intermittently. This has been both a frustration and a feeling of security. Each time I come back to practicing, I find I bring new skills such as organization and communication. I find they enhance my practice. That always increases my respect for the profession of dental hygiene. I feel confident in my skills and that provides a strong sense of security. However, *The Challenger* needs new mountains to climb. Hence, the frustration.

At the present time, as I am putting together my own business, I feel a sense of satisfaction and excitement. It appears that my experience is blending together into an entity that will allow me to use all my skills in a unique way. I will have control over my professional development.

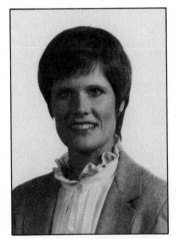

Phebe Blitz

[Phebe is now president of Phebe Blitz and Associates, a professional development team. Her company provides seminars and consulting services for dental health professionals. Contact her at 118 W. Jeanine Drive, Tempe, AZ 85284, 602/839-8856]

Clarify Your Job with an Employment Agreement

The American Dental Hygienists' Association has developed the following sample employment agreement to help both full- and part-time RDHs in private practice establish a stable and equitable business relationship with their dentist employers.

The agreement is not a finished contract. It is a model for both employee and employer to use for expressing their respective needs. Such a document not only clarifies the work relationship, it minimizes the possibility of future misunderstandings.

All elements essential to a valid contract are covered, i.e. which services are to be performed, when and where, the specific method of compensation, and the term (length of time) the agreement is valid.

For additional in-depth guidelines to employment, contact the ADHA, 444 N. Michigan Ave., Suite 3400, Chicago, IL 60611. Tel. 312/440-8900.

ADHA SAMPLE EMPLOYMENT AGREEMENT

THIS AGREEMENT IS MADE THIS ＿＿ day of ＿＿＿＿＿, 19 ＿＿,

＿＿＿＿＿＿＿＿＿＿＿＿＿＿＿＿＿＿＿＿＿＿＿＿＿＿＿

between ＿＿＿＿＿＿＿＿＿＿＿＿and ＿＿＿＿＿＿＿＿＿＿＿＿
             (Dentist)   (Dental Hygienist)

WHEREAS, the Dental Hygienist is a duly licensed (registered) dental hygienist in the State of ＿＿＿＿＿＿＿＿＿ and the parties are desirous of entering into an employment agreement on the terms and conditions hereinafter set forth:

IT IS THEREFORE AGREED AS FOLLOWS:

1. The Dentist hereby employs the Dental Hygienist effective

＿＿＿＿＿＿＿, to perform the services of a Dental Hygienist in the

dental offices at ＿＿＿＿＿＿＿＿＿＿＿＿＿＿＿＿＿＿＿, which
                                (Address)

services shall be consistent with the provisions of the Dental Practice Act of the State of _____, and shall include:

_____

_____

_____

and the Dental Hygienist hereby accepts such employment and agrees to perform the foregoing services in a professional manner. Assignment of additional responsibility is subject to the provisions of paragraph 2.

2. When not performing the services described in paragraph 1, the Dental Hygienist shall perform such other services consistent with the position as may be required from time to time by the Dentist, subject to instructions, direction and supervision of the Dentist, provided that any such services are first described in writing and are performed during the hours and at the place of employment herein stated. The Dental Hygienist shall be paid such additional compensation as may be agreed upon between the parties prior to undertaking the additional services.

3. For the services rendered by the Dental Hygienist described in paragraph 1, the Dentist shall pay to the Dental Hygienist:

Fixed Salary: A Salary of $ _____ per year payable in equal bi-monthly installments of $ _____ each on the _____ and _____ days of each month (a salary of $ _____ per month) such sum to be paid in equal installments of $ _____ on Friday of each week:

Per Diem: A salary at the rate of $ _____ per day (or any fraction thereof) for the days of service actually devoted by the Dental Hygienist to the business of the Dentist which shall be at least _____ days per week (month) payable on the last day of each month).

Per Hour: A salary at the rate of $ _____ per hour (or any fraction thereof) for the hours of service actually devoted by the Dental Hygienist to the business of the Dentist which shall be at least _____ hours per week, payable on the _____ and _____ of each month (payable on Friday of each week).

81

Commission Per Patient: A salary at the rate of $ _____ (a salary based upon a percentage of gross billing) for services rendered per patient treated by the Dental Hygienist, as hereinafter set forth, payable on the _____ and _____ day of each month (payable on the last day of each month):

Services Rendered	Amount (Percentage)
_____	_____
_____	_____
_____	_____

5. The Dental Hygienist shall work _____ days per week for a total of _____ hours per week actually devoted to the practice of dental hygiene provided that such work will not be in excess of _____ hours per day and shall be between the hours of _____ a.m. and _____ p.m. with one hour off for lunch.

6. Whenever required by the nature of the services being performed at that time, the Dental Hygienist shall work for such additional time in any one day beyond the specified _____ hours as may be required, not to exceed _____ hours per day, for which additional services the Dental Hygienist shall receive additional compensation equal to one and one-half times the regular salary agreed to be paid under paragraph 3 of this agreement.

7. The Dental Hygienist shall devote the entire time during the hours specified to the services identified herein and shall be at the place of business of the Dentist during the hours specified.

8. All equipment, supplies and instruments necessary to the proper performance by the Dental Hygienist of the services identified herein are to be provided and paid for by the Dentist.

9. Six months after the effective date of this Agreement, the Dental Hygienist shall be entitled to a paid vacation of _____ business days duration, at a time to be agreed upon by the parties, in an amount for each day of vacation equal to average daily earnings during the thirty working days preceding the vacation. For each six months of work after the first six months, the Dental Hygienist shall be entitled to a paid vacation of _____ days.

10. One month after the effective date of this Agreement, the Dental Hygienist shall be entitled to annual sick leave not to exceed one day per month, which can (cannot) be accumulated in excess of ten (twelve) days.

Other absences, such as funeral leave, personal days, educational session days, etc. will be accrued by the Dentist and the Dental Hygienist.

The Dentist agrees to provide the Dental Hygienist with her/his full pay, whenever the dental hygienist is required to lose a regularly scheduled working day because the dentist is away and/or closes the office. If the Dental Hygienist is unable to work for a longer period of time due to closure of the office by the Dentist (e.g., Dentist's vacation), the Dental Hygienist shall be entitled to her full pay unless the parties have previously agreed to schedule their vacations simultaneously.

11. The Dentist agrees to provide the Dental Hygienist with the following additional employee benefits:

     _____

     _____

     _____

12. Periodic evaluation of the Dental Hygienist's professional performance and review of the compensation provisions described in paragraph 3 will be undertaken by the Dentist with the Dental Hygienist no less frequently than once each year.

13. The term of employment of the Dental Hygienist shall be one year from the date of this Agreement which shall be automatically renewed from year to year hereafter unless terminated by either party upon thirty days written notice prior to expiration of the term of the Agreement. The foregoing notwithstanding, this Agreement shall be terminable without cause of any reason whatsoever by either party upon thirty days prior written notice to the other; provided, that if terminated without cause by Dentist, Dental Hygienist shall be entitled to such compensation as may be due at time of termination plus payment for any vacation time to which she is then entitled.

14. In the event that either party violates any of the provisions of this Agreement, or fails to maintain a license or certificate of registration to practice in this State, then, upon notice of the other party, this Agreement shall at once terminate and neither party shall be under any further obligation to the other except that the Dentist shall pay to the Dental Hygienist such compensation as may be due up to the time of such termination.

IN WITNESS WHEREOF, the parties hereto have signed this Agreement in duplicate on the day and year first above-written.

_____

(DENTIST)

_____

(DENTAL HYGIENIST)

Retail Dentistry

"Retail Dentistry": Friend or Foe?

The words alone often trigger an image of a dental delivery systen performing second-rate dentistry at bargain prices. The reason is that traditional private practitioners cannot understand how a large operation can survive economically without a "quick 'n dirty" approach to patient care.

Once the emotional smokescreen is cleared away, you will find the term "retail dentistry" describes an *approach to the marketing of services*—not a definition of the services themselves.

Key features of this approach are heavy advertising, convenient hours for the patients and commercial locations. The phrase is generally used as a catchall to explain a gamut of dentist-owned operations ranging from practices housed in large retail stores (the first one was in a California Sears), those occupying free-standing retail space in shopping malls or strip shopping centers, to those which otherwise are considered traditional private practices but use retail-type management and marketing techniques.

Some are independently-owned and operated facilities, some are branches of chains, still others are franchises. Many multi-practice retailers are small regional operations while others operate a large number of practices in a variety of geographical settings. All have one thing in common: *They go out of their way to make it as easy as possible for patients to use their services.*

How do they do this? In several ways: they do all the paperwork involved in third party reimbursement, they accept popular credit cards (many of those housed in department stores also accept cards issued by those stores), and perhaps most important, *they are there when the patient—any patient—needs them.* Early morning, late at night, Saturdays, often Sundays, usually holidays, fully staffed.

Fee schedules are highly visible and they make a point of discussing the total cost of any treatment plan before proceeding. (Interestingly, the difference between the fees of a retail dental practice and a traditional practice is rather small, especially for common operative procedures.) *What they do do exceptionally well is de-mystify dentistry.*

Though a primary objective of a retail dental practice is to go after the 50 percent of the population who do not see a dentist regularly, their continued success is dependent on building a good reputation so as to attract all kinds of new patients. And why do these new patients—not just the walk-ins—come? Reasons offered are 1) convenience; 2) dissatisfactions with their previous dentist; 3) no long-term attachment to any dentist; 4) favorable payment policies.

The question of *quality* in retail store practices is based on the same factors dictating quality in a traditional practice: *the individual practitioner's values, abilities and ethics.*

Now, what does all this mean to RDHs? As with any other practice, *retail dentistry cannot survive without a core of patients who make regular preventive visits.*

Most retail practices encourage an identification with the practice rather than with an individual dentist. This can mean that *the RDH is the most regular and recognizable contact the patient has with the practice.* Opportunities for RDHs lie not only in exercising their clinical expertise, but in using their educational abilities (frequently patients come to the practice with low dental IQ's) and in developing their supervisory, marketing, public relations and practice management skills. In short, a good way to expand and broaden one's career in dental hygiene.

Word of mouth will tell you where retail dental centers are in your area. And so will the local radio station, the neighborhood shopper and the ads in the Yellow Pages. Chances are your neighborhood mall has one.

New modalities always bring with them the critics of change and the status quo. But they also bring interesting and exciting challenges for those who see opportunity.

RDH in a Dental Center

Kathleen Somers discusses her feelings in letting go of one opportunity to move into another dimension of dental health care.

Overcoming Burnout

I have been a hygienist since 1973. Up until the middle of 1984, I worked full time in a small private practice. It is a good practice and my employer was and is a sweet, easygoing person. After seven years, however, my goals, ambitions and financial need began to overshadow the comfort of a practice where everything became so routine that boredom and burnout began to take its toll.

At first I fought these feelings by becoming more active in the association component in which I have been an active member since graduation. I also began working on my bachelor's degree through an external degree program. This program allows flexibility in amassing credits by courses offered at area colleges, correspondence courses, credit by examination, and demonstration of subject knowledge by portfolio. My degree, (the name of which was new to me), will be called Bachelor of Science in Dental Hygienics. I will have my minor in business management.

Doing this helped relieve my discontent for a while. I also had the feeling that I owed my employer some great debt because he "gave" me my first dental hygiene job. This, in spite of the fact that I only went on *one* interview—his—for a dental hygiene position!

Then, I switched my alliance to owing "my" patients. After all, I had cared and been responsible for them for a long time and considered them friends. How could I leave them?

What could I do about my feelings? How do I give myself permission to know I also owe myself?

During this time, I began to feel I needed to run away from dentistry —the faster and farther the better. I was beginning to see the physical and mental effects of stress and burnout. What do I do? I wondered. Being self-supporting, I had fixed expenses and could not just walk away without another position. So I stayed.

I began a fruitless search for a career change. I had two associate degrees and great credentials but no four-year degree and no management or supervisory experience necessary to make a complete career change.

Finally, I admitted to myself what several career counselors, friends, and personnel department heads had told me: build on what you have. That, for me, meant dental experience and continuing with my educational goals. I would get that four-year degree! For a job change, I started to look in the dental section of the classified ads getting myself ready to answer them mentally.

Opportunity Appears

At a spring association meeting, the invited speaker was a periodontist/owner of a large group practice in the area. He presented a professional picture which conflicted with my biased vision of a dental center's patient population and standards of practice.

During the meeting he casually mentioned that his Center would be needing to add a hygienist to its staff. Two months later, while I was in the area interviewing for positions outside of dentistry. I stopped at the Center, résumé in hand and business suit on.

Luck was with me. Without an appointment I met and spoke with the senior hygienist. My résumé and professional association involvement, as well as my working towards my bachelor's degree impressed my interviewer. So much so that she set up a meeting with the Center's administrator.

At this interview, I was told of plans for a hygiene department. Until that point, the hygiene function had been a poor stepchild of the Center. The owners were now, after four years in business, seeing the need to elevate the hygiene function to its true place in dentistry as an integral part in the Center's goals and mission: to deliver complete and thorough dental care to the patient population for a lifetime.

The administrator was very upbeat regarding the Center's future goals and asked me to accompany the owners, hygienist and office manager to a *Quest Seminar. The Seminar was on how to set up a hygiene department, complete with assistants, if I accepted the position.

My third meeting was with the owners, at which time I stated my goals for myself as they applied to the Center and what I expected from a hygiene program within the Center's structure. Those goals were and are: to progress away from prophy after prophy, to utilize my abilities and expanded functions license, to be able to learn from the

*Practice management seminars for dental offices, specializing in information and skills necessary for the creation of accelerated dental practices and dental hygiene departments.

91

different specialists and general dentists, to involve myself in the marketing of dentistry, and, most important, to become an integral part of the hygiene department with a high probability of managerial and supervisory duties.

The doctor-owners agreed (with some modifications) and offered an hourly salary plus bonus for production along with nine personal days, 10 vacation days and 50 percent payment of a group major medical insurance program and overtime pay based on time and a half.

Continuing education courses are paid 50 to 100 percent depending on the course. The salary range for an RDH was $10.00 to $12.36 an hour, and for an expanded functions RDH such as myself was $11.00 to $13.50. I am, in my state, licensed as "dental hygienist specialist." This means I can do expanded duties in addition to dental hygiene. I could choose my hours, but two evenings per week and alternating Saturdays were required since these are prime-time hours for our patients.

How I Made My Decision

I had given myself time after each interview to think about the pros and cons of the position. I believe I made 90 percent of my decision based on the second interview for the following reasons:

(1) The administrator assured me that the hygiene department was an immediate goal of the Center's plan.

(2) I would have the opportunity to meet, work with and learn from other professionals. (This was not possible in a smaller practice environment.)

(3) The potential to grow into a management position was as great as the probability of the hygiene department.

(4) I felt there was genuine sincerity since I was asked to attend the *Quest Seminar* even before I was to begin my association with the Center.

(5) Having an administrator on staff gave me the confidence that the Center was indeed a corporate structure, not just a large group practice.

(6) There were good benefits, salary, and flexiblity of hours, despite the evenings required, plus a total of 19 days off per year.

The disadvantages I saw were leaving a shorter work schedule and going from familiar to uncertain surroundings. The pros far outweighed the cons.

A larger setting, potential for management, a substantial increase in salary and benefits, and the change I needed at this time were more important. I also felt that being in the larger corporate setting might open doors to other opportunities.

And so, after my third interview, I made my decision. I called within 24 hours with my salary requirements and redefined the responsibilities of the position and the hours.

Within the week, I received a formal proposal with the salary I had asked for. I accepted the proposal by formal letter restating all the conditions.

Progress Report

After six months, I have no regrets, although the hygiene department is not quite yet a reality. We have had several meetings as to the structure, placement of the additional operatories, whose jurisdiction the assistants would be under, etc.

My aim is to have the hygiene department responsible for its budget, supplies, equipment, and personnel leading to total department fiscal responsibility within the Center's structure.

Clinical responsibilities will include preliminary assessment and treatment planning, treating all oral conditions which fall within the scope of expanded functions dental hygiene practice, and providing complete and thorough prophylaxis and patient education services. The patient's dentist will examine and finalize all treatment plans. The hygiene department will coordinate efforts of the professional and office support staff to insure complete client care.

What the Center Is

The Center is not, by ADA definition, "retail dentistry." It is a free-standing structure with its own separate entrances adjacent to two nationally-known department stores in a large shopping mall; independently owned and separate from any other corporation or franchise.

The physical appearance is very pleasing. Art work is placed in common areas and each operatory has a scenic mural to enjoy. The Center shares the services of the Mall Association regarding such things as security and outside maintenance. The Center is open 73 hours per week (coinciding with those of the mall), except Sundays. Appointments are necessary other than for emergencies.

At the present time, hygiene appointments are scheduled for thirty minutes with the option to reappoint for those patients who need more care or to refer the patient to the proper specialist. The hygiene time is totally devoted to education and prophys. The exam is done prior to or just after the hygiene appointment by the patient's dentist.

The patient population is well educated and has a mid-to-high dental IQ. The patient pool includes professionals, middle managers, white-collar employees, educators, and trades people. Financially, they are primarily in the mid-socioeconomic range. Better than fifty percent of them are covered by dental insurance through their employers.

How I Feel Now

Did I make the right decision to leave a small, two-operatory private practice to go into a large, 16-operatory dental center? For me, the answer is yes. This setting permits me more potential for growth, clinically and professionally, both within the Center and for future career opportunities. It has also given me more economic freedom.

What advice would I give to an RDH interested in such a work environment? Find out if there is a full-time administrator. This offers a more business-like setting. When you have a problem, there is someplace to take it, be listened to, and resolved.

Talk to the other hygienists on staff to find out if the center lives up to their commitments to a staff and to patients. Visit the center so that if you do have any negative thoughts about such facilities they will be dispelled.

Enjoy your right to negotiate for yourself. Give yourself permission.

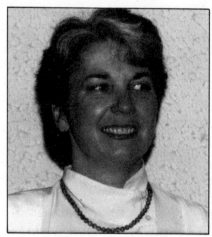

Kathleen Somers

Operational Prepaid Health Care Plans in the United States

Health Maintenance Organizations

Q. What is a health maintenance organization?

A. A health maintenance organization (HMO) is a managed health care plan that provides or arranges for the delivery of comprehensive, coordinated medical services to voluntarily enrolled members on a prepaid basis.

Q. How do they operate?

A. There are three basic model types of HMOs:

1) A *group practice model* delivers services at one or more locations through a group of doctors who contract with the HMO to provide care;

2) A *staff model* delivers services through doctors who are employees of the HMO and who also practice collectively from one or more facilities;

3) An *individual practice association* (IPA) makes contractual arrangements with doctors in the community to provide health services to HMO members out of their own offices.

In addition to the three basic model types, there are *network* HMOs which contract with two or more group practices to provide health services.

Q. Which type is the most popular?

A. IPA models account for over 51 percent of all operational HMOs. Most dental groups fall in that category, an example being a dentist who has contracted with a union or other organization to provide dental services in his own office. Co-payment by the patient is often required.

Q. Where do you find these HMOs?

A. Forty-three states, the District of Columbia and Guam have at least one HMO, 35 states and the District of Columbia have five or more, and 21 states have 10 or more HMOs (ex: California, Michigan, New York).

Q. Who finances them, besides the members?

A. The federal government in part, but the majority reflect investments from the private sector. There are currently 14 major chains representing both for-profit and non-profit HMOs. Some, like the Prudential and CIGNA insurance companies, develop, manage and own their HMOs. Others, like HealthAmerica and Blue Cross/Blue Shield, provide a combination of management services and ownership among their affiliated plans. And still others, such as Charter Med and Hancock/Dikewood, provide management services through a contractual basis.

Q. Do a lot of people belong? Do they like them?

A. Over 21 million people are now enrolled in approximately 480 plans—almost four times the number of members enrolled a decade ago. At this rate of growth, some experts feel that as much as half of the enrolled population may receive their health care from managed care systems by the mid-1990's.

Consumer acceptance is measured by enrollment. In Minneapolis, for example, where only two percent of the population belonged to an HMO ten years ago, 26 percent belong today.

The reasons cited for joining an HMO are lower costs, availability to doctors, preventive health services, and comprehensive benefits.

Q. Do all HMOs have dental components?

A. It has been estimated that less than 25 percent of established HMOs offer dental services. However, there has been an increase in the IPA networking model among private practitioners.

Q. Where can I get more information?

A. If working in an HMO appeals to you, why not initiate discussion with the people running them? This starts you "networking" with decision makers whom you can then ask to keep you informed. Changes often occur without a great deal of fanfare and a program may be in its beginning stages. You could be getting in on the ground floor of the dental program!

Health Maintenance Organizations are generally listed in the Yellow Pages. As for IPA dental practices, call your state dental association to see if they have any data on which dental practices are IPA models.

(Most of the preceding information was extrapolated from publications of the Health Care Financing Administration, Dept. of Health & Human Services.)

For additional information on HMOs contact:

Office of Health Maintenance Organizations
Department of Health & Human Services
5600 Fishers Lane
Rockville, MD 20857

Group Health Association of America
624 Ninth Street, N.W.
Washington, D.C. 20001

American Medical Care and Review Association
5410 Grosvenor Lane, Suite 210
Bethesda, MD 20814

RDH in a
Health Maintenance
Organization

Mary Ellen Winner *discusses her shift from private practice to an alternate care setting.*

I graduated from dental hygiene school over thirty years ago, worked a year, married, moved to Pennsylvania, worked some more, then started our family thinking that I would probably never work as a full-time RDH again. Wrong!

Three children and 18 years later my husband became very ill and the prognosis was devastating. I was advised to start looking for a position, yet was not licensed in the state in which we resided.

Miraculously, there was a local dental hygiene school offering a refresher course. With tremendous support and aid from my family, I was able to enroll in the course, study, take the Boards and pass successfully.

I had a lot to work out after my husband died. Now to support our family. In searching for a job, I mentioned to my friend, "wouldn't it be good if a position opened up because the hygienist became pregnant." The very next week there was such an ad in the newspaper!

I applied for the job, was interviewed and offered the position. I accepted and stayed with that practice for 11 years, working in other offices on Saturdays.

Volunteering

During this period, I returned to college for my associate's degree and began my volunteer activities. Volunteering is a tremendous learning experience as well as a way of meeting many fabulous people. The interchange between colleagues, like any position in life, is beautiful, enlightening, challenging, exhausting—and fun!

When I joined the ADHA, I volunteered to be the employment chairperson, developing salary and benefit surveys. Eventually I became co-treasurer of the state association, designing improved bookkeeping methods and standards for disbursements. I thoroughly enjoyed those four years.

Shifting Goals

Then my daughter-in-law became extremely ill. My son and his wife belonged to a health maintenance organization, commonly referred to as an HMO. Her illness contributed toward a change of my thinking and goals at this period of my life.

I truly believe that one of the reasons my daughter-in-law is alive today is due to the *caring attitude* of the employees and the *total care* she received at their HMO.

Fortunately, the supervisor of the dental component was a friend of mine. She was looking for additional hygienists to fill in when full-time staff took vacation or personal days. I began working there.

At first I was swamped by all the paperwork. It seemed to be so immense—so many different forms, so different from private practice! But I soon became accustomed to it all.

The Setting

Working in an HMO is similar to private practice, yet different. The dentists can concentrate on dentistry without the everyday business hassles. This is evident in the almost stressfree atmosphere.

The goals of the group model open panel HMO, such as the one I'm in, are to provide comprehensive health care to an enrolled population for a fixed monthly rate.

We are prevention oriented, have a diversity of patients of all ages, some of whom have never had dental treatment. We can automatically refer patients for perio, endo or oral surgery treatment if needed. The interplay between medical and dental, especially for referrals to lab testing, medication for existing conditions, or to the nutritionist is right there. We have a supervisor for help in problem-solving, and ongoing staff meetings, some with the specialists who give mini-seminars. An exciting atmosphere, to be sure.

Opportunity Calls

A full-time position was posted. I applied for it, was accepted, and began traveling to three different centers (all under the same umbrella.) I felt as if I were working three different jobs: learning the drawer systems, developing time-motion operations for six different operatories, interacting with staff. It was a challenge!

I began to be comfortable with the work habits of each of the five full-time and one part-time dentists, the five full-time and two part-time hygienists and other staff members. Everyone at the centers is supportive and there for each other. It is a nice atmosphere.

At the present time, I'm only going to two centers plus working with the periodontist one day a week. (In this particular HMO, the RDH working with the periodontist is paid $2.00 more per patient—an added incentive.)

101

Salaries and Benefits

At this time, 1987, the hourly salary range for RDHs in my HMO is from over eleven dollars to not quite eighteen. If this seems on the small side, remember that the benefits package is better than the community average, totaling 35 percent of salary.

Annual benefits include paid holidays, personal days, sick time, tuition reimbursement, bereavement leave, complete health insurance with a no-pay prescription card. There is a dental discount of 50 percent, life and disability insurance, malpractice insurance, and I even get to pick my own vacation times! But I must stress that I did not leave private practice for the benefits package, great as it is. It was the delivery system and concept which appealed to me.

One of the biggest negatives to this story is that I miss all those beautiful private practice patients: the complete families, toddlers and great-grandparents that I knew. It isn't easy to build up "private patients" in an HMO, especially when you are scheduled in different centers.

Another problem I experienced initially related to instrument usage. Everyone has a different concept of "what's sharp." After stating the problem to the supervisor, she had me order my own set-ups. That took care of the problem.

A Typical Day

If I am working a morning/afternoon shift, I usually arrive at work at least 30 minutes early. Why? Because there is a lot to be done and there's little last-minute time to do it.

Everyone likes to set up the operatory according to one's own methods. I like to rewipe the equipment, review charts, insert the dental sheets, health histories, forms....If there's been a change in the schedule I must order new charts from the Records Department. All these things take precious time and I don't want to take away from patient care time to do them.

The morning session usually involves five patients, the afternoon session, four. The exception to this is when I work as co-therapist with the periodontist. Then only four patients are scheduled in the morning.

Generally 45 minutes are allotted for each patient. I often run over as this includes treatment time, patient education, and at least five to ten minutes for paperwork.

Documentation is most important in records. I document parental permission for taking X-rays and giving fluoride treatments. If, when I review the health history, the patient tells me his or her health has changed since the last visit, I document that change, including new medications the patient is taking. If further dental treatment is necessary, the patient is given a treatment plan with fees.

When a cancellation occurs, my time is spent checking equipment to see what needs inspection, maintenance or restocking.

Solving Problems

Being somewhat overwhelmed by the variety of forms forced me to create a "forms" manual for incoming auxiliaries. (This also included examples of the instrument set-ups used by the doctors.)

This, in turn, led to a maintenance manual. In here is information on equipment maintenance, including handpiece and prophy angle care and how to clean the lights on the units.

From these two manuals evolved a posted monthly maintenance chart with designated areas to check off as the daily needs are noted. There are times for each of us when you can't recall having completed a specific task. What with changing shifts, we needed some method of tracking what was being done and when. Now we had it. Next came an improved time-motion flow for infection control, followed by a file for catalogue information.

When I travel, I enjoy visiting other HMOs. It sparks my mind to rethink various aspects of my own work environment.

If it's challenge and variety you want, consider working in a health maintenance organization.

*[Interested readers can contact Mary Ellen Winner through **Career Directions for Dental Hygienists**.]*

How to Turn
Your Volunteer Work
Into a Job

The Benefits of Volunteering

The voluntary or non-profit sector of our society, such as in neighborhood associations, public interest lobbies, self-help or support groups, hospitals, churches or synagogues, nursing homes, not-for-profit agencies, and yes, your professional association, could not exist without unpaid volunteers.

A survey by The Independent Sector, a coalition of several hundred nonprofit organizations, found that 89 million Americans aged 14 and older did some volunteer work in 1985. They averaged at least three and a half hours of volunteering per week. If they had been paid, the bill would have come to $110 billion!

Traditionally, most volunteers were married women who did not work outside the home. However today, not only do men constitute 45% of the voluntary work force, but 57% of married women with children work outside the home. (More than two-thirds of the women between the ages of 25 and 44 are employed.)

These significant facts reveal that professionals, with paying jobs elsewhere and with extremely busy personal lives, are now the fastest-growing segment of the volunteer work force.

Volunteering can be a smart move for RDHs because the opportunities for personal satisfaction, professional growth, and ultimate profit are several. Consider this:

1) *The friends and associates you meet in your volunteer efforts can be part of your networking system.* When the time comes for you to make a career move, let people in your organization know. Since they are already familiar with your level of energy and work habits, you may find someone who knows someone who is looking for someone...

Equally important is the laying of the foundation of a reciprocal professional network. This means establishing your credentials with other professionals who are in the same organization as you.

When your patients require the services of another type of specialist, you do your best to recommend a professional you know can do the job, don't you?

Well, those specialists with whom you have a reciprocal referral system will send patients to you when dental health services such as you perform are required.

2) *Identify your newly-developed skills in your résumé.* Did you set up the booth, get the bodies, make the posters, distribute the fliers for an oral health screening or lobbying effort?

Did you write a spot announcement or publicity release for the local media or for your organization's publication? Have you tabulated the results of a mailing or telephone call-for-donations to recruit money, products or people?

You can now *document* your organizational skills, your public relations training, your administrative capabilities.

Give these accomplishments the dignity of "non-clinical experience" as you construct your résumé. Not being paid for your volunteer work doesn't diminish its worth. Just don't make a point of it.

3) If you've targeted a non-traditional environment for practicing dental hygiene, find out who the director of volunteers is for the program relevant to your goal. Now "sell" that person on what you can do. Once you get the go-ahead, contribute on a limited but regular basis. Make yourself a valuable resource they want to keep coming.

Once you have demonstrated your value, money, often, has a way of appearing. More than one RDH has found her way into a private nursing home, day care center, or handicapped program with this approach.

The down side is that you may be rejected, be told that what you propose isn't needed. Take the case of RDH Phebe Blitz. School administrators rejected her educational proposal claiming that the school nurse was already doing dental health education.

Rather than arguing her case, Phebe handled the situation by saying, "Gee, I'm delighted to hear that such a program is being done! I would like to offer some of my very current educational materials to her for her use."

She then talked with the nurse, found her *most* receptive because her materials *were* outdated. She was thoroughly appreciative of Phebe's help. As Phebe recounts, "Once I got her on my side, the two of us approached another member of the organization and from that point on, the rest was easy."

4) *You will draw people to your office through speaking engagements.* As a result of an effective presentation, you can not only influence the audience but can also motivate people to call you.

The best way to position yourself to be invited to speak to any local organization is, of course, to be a member of that group.

An excellent way to spread the word that you are available for lecturing is to type up a one-page letter explaining who you are and a little about your background. Write a short summary describing three topics which you are prepared to speak on.

Send photocopies of this letter to those community groups you're interested in. Then follow up the letters with phone calls about two or three weeks later. This act will reinforce your interest and serious-ness and should generate some engagements.

When you do speak, remember to hand out literature or business cards that bear your name and/or that of your employer. This way members of the audience will have an easy time contacting you if they wish to do so.

Meeting the Challenge

An unusual approach was effectively used by RDH Jan Shurts. When a dentist complained that Tulsa (Oklahoma) hygienists were unwill-ing to donate time to help the poor, Jan bristled at the remark and rallied members of her local component into volunteer action. The tar-get of their efforts was an organization that ministers to the medical and dental needs of the elderly, disabled, handicapped and the poor.

Designing the hygiene area and corresponding program proved to be Jan's entree into this not-for-profit, non-government subsidized or-ganization run by an ex-priest. When the dental director left, Jan was asked to join the staff in that capacity since she then had so much experience with the program.

Initially, there were two evening clinics with seven dentist volunteers. Through her successful recruiting, Jan now directs the volunteer ef-forts of 35 dentists and 40 auxiliaries to offer five clinics throughout the week.

Because of the visibility that comes from this position, Jan was offered a part-time position with the Indian Health Service where she now also works.

This energetic RDH claims, "I've gotten a long way on an associate's degree, and volunteering in and through my association has proved very valuable to this success."

Earning College Credit for Community Service

Did you know it's possible for your volunteer efforts to earn you credit towards a college degree? Well, according to Susan Simosko, national network coordinator for Project Learn of the Council for Adult and Ex-periential Learning, they can.

CAEL is a non-profit international association of institutions, agen-cies and individuals dedicated to fostering quality learning outside the traditional academic experience. A frequent comment staff often hears is, "Oh! You mean we can get credit for *that*?"

Ms. Simosko's job is to disseminate information nationwide about Project Learn—a national network of information on adult learner services. It is now possible for a learner in one region of the country to have access to a program 2,000 miles away whether it be for an external degree or for a correspondence course.

She points out that Congress has recently passed a law whereby financial aid is now available to part-time students—a milestone for adult education and a boon for financially-strapped dedicated adult learners.

To find out how to evaluate your knowledge so you can turn it into college credit, contact CAEL at 10840 Little Patuxent Pkwy., Suite 203, Columbia, MD 21044. The telephone number for Washington, D.C. residents is 301/596-6799; for all others, 301/997-3535.

Volunteering your time and energy can be valuable training for an RDH, transferable to many different efforts. It is a good opportunity for those eager to demonstrate their ogranizational skills, for those welcoming the chance to be recognized by the broader health care community as the best person to communicate dental health information. Your image will be enhanced.

Rewards will be personal satisfaction, professional growth and, ultimately, profits.

109

What You Need to Know About Owning Your Own Business

The term "managerial strategies" is not a phrase that is in the working vocabulary of most RDHs. It sits awkwardly in the middle of our dental language which, in its own unintended way, often separates us from the non-dental person.

Unfamiliar, perhaps, is a better word than uncomfortable to describe our reaction when we hear that one of our colleagues has "gone into business for herself." We ask ourselves how and where these people acquired the acumen and capital to undertake such a venture.

The first thing you need for starting *any* business is a *business plan.* That becomes your tool for acquiring the necessary capital.

Where To Start

SCORE (Service Corps of Retired Executives) is a non-profit organization of retired business people offering a consulting service at no charge. You can find them on college campuses, public libraries, through notices on bulletin boards in your local post office, or through the Chamber of Commerce. They are good people in whom to confide your ideas without feeling inadequate or foolish. They can help you to organize and center your thinking and objectives.

Another starting point is the U.S. Small Business Administration which provides counseling, training and financial assistance to those interested in starting their own business.

The SBA publishes many booklets on the subject; you might want to start off with *Thinking About Going Into Business?* or *How To Develop a Business Plan.* These booklets are available free from the SBA, P.O. Box 15434, Fort Worth, TX 76119, or your nearest SBA office (listed under "United States Government" in your telephone book).

According to the founder of American Woman's Economic Development Corp (AWED), women who venture into their own businesses have a lower failure rate than men. Why? Because women seem to evidence an "extraordinary commitment" to make the business successful. However, they often have no background in skills like pricing, accounting, marketing.

For a $35 fee, women can buy up to 90 minutes of time talking on the phone with business experts. By calling AWED's toll-free number 1-800-222-AWED (212-692-9100 in New York), women can make an appointment with business counselors and AWED calls them back at AWED's expense.

Regardless of what type of business you go into, you'll have to decide what legal form of organization to use. Here are some details about two major forms, along with the major rewards and drawbacks.

• *Sole Proprietorship.* This is the most common form a start-up business takes. As sole owner, you control the business and take all the profits, which are lumped with other personal income and taxed accordingly. You may offset business losses against your personal income.

No legal formalities are required, and it's easy to start up or close down the business. Bookkeeping, tax and legal problems generally are relatively simple.

The greatest drawback is that you are responsible for all debts, and your personal assets can be at risk. That liability puts a limit on the amount of capital you can borrow, so expansion may depend largely on reinvested profits. You also may find it harder to attract and keep key employees who may want an ownership stake.

• *Partnership.* This consists of two or more owners, perhaps including general (managing) and limited partners (investors). One advantage of a partnership is that more people can invest in the business, using personal assets as collateral for loans. They may also contribute expertise to various aspects of running the enterprise.

Partners are taxed in the same way as sole proprietors, and general partners are both individually and collectively liable for the partnership's debts and other partners' actions.

Unless you and your partners get along, the arrangement may make everyone miserable. If one partner dies or withdraws from the business, the partnership is terminated. The other partners may then have to buy out that partner's share or find a buyer who wants to become a partner.

In short, there's a lot of homework to be done before you start your own business. You've got to learn what it takes to make a business run and what sort of market exists for the services you want to provide.

Three Who Did It

Planning sets the tone for future business success. It is to this planning, vision, dedication and integrity that each of the following RDH business owners speaks.

If there is a common thread linking these impressive and accomplished women, it is that they bring to their businesses hard work, self-discipline, and an enormous desire to control their own destinies. But never by compromising their value systems or rejecting their profession.

113

Each has set about attaining her goals by design, by plan, and by understanding that success is built on method, time, and the hopscotch of alternative directions and decisions. Plus the confidence to believe one isn't a failure if success is not achieved overnight.

Risk-takers? Perhaps. Competent and determined professionals? Yes.

RDH as Personnel Placement Agency Owner

Katherine Simons *describes her evolution into owning her own business.*

Balance. For me the very word conjures up images of sleepless nights full of problem solving, lazy summer Sunday afternoons floating on Atlanta's Lake Lanier, hot meals on the table, living with challenging teenage daughters, and the excitement of turning a business concept into a virtual necessity for so many of our doctors.

Balance is the struggle of wanting to have it all succeed and knowing when each area requires that extra effort, the extra push, thought and drive. It means staying in tune, being in touch, following through to the end . . . stretching the possibilities.

And so, at age 40—itself an age for reflection—I view my life with its many roles as a delicate blending of needs and wishes, while taking all things into consideration with each change.

Starting Out

As a young woman growing up in a family of four in a suburb of New York City, I had a consistent and involved church life. As far back as I can remember, one element of my life was always clear: my life's purpose was to be in service. I knew financial reward would come.

Service has taken on many different faces at different times. My first career choice was nursing. Off I went to college. A summer in a dental office and pending marriage plans put a halt to that direction. Dental assisting and becoming a wife then brought with it a whole new set of opportunities.

During the three years I was an assistant, I began to look into ways of increasing my knowledge of dentistry. I knew the mechanics, but the "whys" of each function were not always clear.

I discovered that a dental hygiene education would allow me to know the "whys" and also give me the opportunity to produce results from my efforts by working directly in the patient's mouth.

I realized that depending on what I knew, how I utilized my skills, and how I motivated the patients, I could produce results that would make a real difference in the health of another human being. My husband graduated from college that June; I began the dental hygiene program the following September.

115

After Graduation

I was employed full time at first and then part time after my two daughters were born. Fortunately, I did not have to work to keep a roof over our heads or food on the table. I could choose to pursue the difficult, challenging and rewarding task of mothering and home care.

Once again, balance was important. I felt a need to continue to develop my professional knowledge and skills. I found the answer in practicing hygiene one day a week while participating in the local dental hygiene association.

When the girls were both in elementary school, I felt the time had come to begin developing my career. In talking with other RDHS, I discovered a lot of dissatisfaction. This discovery greatly influenced my decisions about my own career path. I realized that whatever my direction, I would probably need a bachelor's degree.

The Right Move

I enrolled in a non-traditional degree program designed for those who had already completed an associate degree in a technical field such as nursing or dental hygiene. The high concentration of social service courses were so fascinating to me that I considered rechoosing my career path.

Except for a very wise instructor, I may have entered social services. During a class, I wrote a paper about changing career directions. My instructor advised me to incorporate my experiences into my already present knowledge base. It was wonderful advice and I followed it.

Change is wonderful and important. Don't be afraid of it. Change is growth. Coupled with careful planning and research, it can bring large rewards.

Identifying Needs

The dissatisfaction I heard from practicing hygienists and dental assistants became louder in my ears. The communication skills I learned through the social work classes opened many doors. New ways for me to serve in my chosen field became apparent. I began to see the unrest in offices as a result of mismatched goals, skills and personalities. For example, I would often find dental assistants lacking a clear sense of purpose in the services they were performing.

As the need became clearer, so did the result. The dental community needed a way to match dental staff with dentists. Dental staff needed a place for ongoing learning about the "whys" behind excellent dental care. They needed education in radiograph placement, sterilization techniques, and the "how-tos" of expanded duties.

The result would be dental *professionals* with a renewed sense of purpose and greater self-confidence. A new and valuable service could be offered to increase satisfaction for both doctor and staff.

In addition, new career opportunities could develop where they didn't exist before. Thus, the beginning of a new career direction for me and the birth of a new service in Atlanta, Georgia.

Making it Happen

The next step was developing a plan, a support system, networking, and learning how to be a business owner. My husband has written business plans for years. He wrote a detailed plan for what was to be called **Dynamic Dental Services (D.D.S.).**

He carefully formulated projections which detailed each progressive step re expenses vs. income and the level of business needed to support continued growth.

Later I had a marketing plan professionally written which outlined a tailored approach to get from point A to *result* Z. Time lines were formulated and specific plans made to achieve desired results.

Dynamic Dental Services has become Atlanta's primary source for staffing, résumé critiques, referrals, personnel forms, sharing of ideas among the dental community and continuing education, as well as a sounding board for dentists and staff alike.

My Continued Professional Growth

Part of the marketing plan included personal development for me. Seminars and workshops provided by private companies were suggested as part of my professional growth.

I have listened to tapes, attended intensive workshops on public speaking, interpersonal relations and leadership skills. I maintain membership and board positions with several professional associations. I feel I have begun to fill my need for giving service to my profession and my community.

The Circle Comes Around

Once again, I am looking at creating sufficient balance in my life. I am married 20 years, have two teenage daughters, my business is now three years old.

All these changes have created many adjustments. There constantly need to be checkpoints, evaluations, and shifts in behavior to assure that family and health needs are being met. I find that having written goals and making planned, careful changes and shifts in direction assists me in making these changes less stressful.

On Change

Helen Keller has stated, "When one door of happiness closes, another opens, but often we look so long at the closed door that we do not see the one which has opened for us."

Yes, changing career directions is certainly stressful. However, careful planning and balancing our priorities at each step along the way are the key elements to both enjoying the challenge and keeping our eyes on the open door.

I am now thankful that I chose to develop my career based on my existing knowledge and experience.

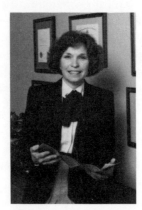

Katherine Simons

*[Readers can contact Katherine Simons at **Dynamic Dental Services, Inc.,** 1175 Grimes Bridge Rd., Suite 302, Roswell, GA 30075. Tel. 404/998-7779]*

RDH as Seminar Promoter

Marsha Raff *began her business of promoting seminars for health care professionals through her volunteer activities.*

"Would you be our continuing education chairman for the year?" I was asked. Little did I realize that accepting this position for the San Francisco dental hygiene component eight years after graduating with my bachelor's degree would be the first step towards my own continuing education business years later.

I was never a leader or gung-ho organization person during my high school or college years. In fact, I was so tired of the educational setting by the time I finally reached my goal of being a hygienist, that it was years until I even felt like attending a seminar.

I accepted the position of continuing education chairman as a favor to my friend who was president that year. She said, "You really don't have to plan anything, if you don't want to. Nobody else ever has." You see, continuing education wasn't mandatory in California at that time so there was very little interest in it.

One thing I had learned about myself in life was that it gives me great pleasure to take something that has attracted little attention in the past and make a big splash with it. I decided to plan one spectacular continuing education seminar for our component and advertise it to the rest of Northern California!

I went to the dental department of an army hospital and organized a course utilizing their facilities and army personnel from all parts of the U.S., most of it at their expense. This ended up being an annual event for the next three years. (During one of these years I was president of our component.)

The Work Involved

It didn't take long for me to recognize there were a hundred and one details involved in planning a continuing education seminar. Choosing a popular topic was only the first step. I would later realize that all the principles that apply to the functioning of any large business are there, EVERY ONE OF THEM, even in the planning of one seminar!

I worked with separate companies that sold labels, designed and printed the brochure, and mailed out the brochures. Then there were differences in dealing with the facilities, whether it was a hotel, school or conference center. Within that category, coordination was necessary with caterers and audiovisual experts. Detail work included handling incoming applications and checks, keeping accurate accounting of expenses, sending confirmation letters, and dealing with incoming calls for information.

Rewards for me came on the day of the course when I would receive praise for a job well done. Inside, I felt creative. I knew that many hygienists had furthered their education as a result of my efforts, and that I had an opportunity to personally interact with many stimulating business people. Looking back now, I know that I was gaining first-hand, on-the-job skills and training that could be used in the future. (And that would be difficult to duplicate, even in a business class!)

For the next three years I was continuing education chairperson for the Northern California State Dental Hygiene Association. My responsibilities were to offer guidance to all the component continuing education chairpersons with any courses they had planned. I also planned numerous association-sponsored courses for the general membership.

The fact that no income was produced from my many hours involved in continuing education was acceptable to me. I was happily married at the time and did not require extra money. I worked at hygiene full time for five years after school, but not at all during this particular period.

Obstacles to Overcome

My life and financial situation abruptly changed when my husband left me and I was faced with raising my one-and four-year-old sons alone. This situation demanded an immediate source of income. Although two days per week at hygiene wasn't sufficient, it was all I could manage with the balancing act necessary between my hectic household and the stresses inherent in coping with an unexpected divorce.

When call after call to me was, "Since you aren't putting on courses any longer nothing's worth attending," a hygienist friend and I decided to begin our own continuing education business. Timing in one's life is crucial. In 1977 there were no continuing education providers in Northern California (other than the two dental schools) and continuing education had just become mandatory. The field was wide open. With a very small investment to purchase a list of name labels, my colleague and I mailed our first course brochure. We received 130 responses.

During the next few years—not knowing any better—we did no advance planning. We would promote one seminar per brochure, collect our profits and then rush to get something else together. We didn't know the meaning of long-range planning and if we had been asked what our goals were, we would have drawn a blank. We hadn't even speculated as to where all of this could lead.

Little by little, however, we began to take risks, each of which could have been disasterous enough to wipe out our finances. Even though we often had over 200 participants at each seminar, we were charging very little. And this included gourmet lunches! After a while the realization sets in that even though all this work is fun in the beginning, there comes a time when you have to treat it like a business and earn a reasonable amount for the time spent. We started planning.

By listing several course descriptions on one brochure to save on postage, increasing our mailing to assistants and dentists, and eliminating most of the lunches, we were beginning to operate more intelligently. Soon competition was everywhere and we had to work harder to promote our courses.

After three years, my partner left the business and I've continued alone for an additional four years. My lenient employer allowed me to conduct business calls between patients and on my lunch hour. In addition, I worked every day and most evenings as well as weekends when the seminars took place. I was constantly trying out new ideas in an effort to expand the business.

By now there was a pattern to my mailings and I was trying seminars out-of-state and out of the U.S. You can never stop thinking of new ideas. The seminars you plan always have to be on the most current subjects and offer more than that of your competitors.

Pros and Cons

What advice would I give those interested in entering this business? At this time, the upfront costs and committments are considerable and there's no guarantee that the program you're sponsoring will be a money-maker. What may be a success one time can flop the next. People tend to see only the well-attended courses and count the profits. They don't understand the hidden costs of running a business.

Also, there is no assurance of a set salary you can count on. You have to be able to deal with that as well as the stresses and a disruptive schedule if you are working out of your home, as I do. Amazing problems can occur at any time, from a speaker who is in a plane crash and can't appear, to a slide projector that breaks down with the speaker refusing to go on without one.

However, for me the benefits offset the liabilities. I like having flexible hours, knowing that I have complete control over what I do, and being able to take ideas and carry them through to the end. I have been amazed to learn time and again that I can cope with challenging situations and come out the better for it. Many of my closest friends are people I have met through the business. My biggest reward has always been seeing how enthusiastic and highly-motivated the attendees are by the end of a seminar.

Financially, if you average out the seminars, the income probably equals dental hygiene pay on a yearly basis, but less if you break this down into an hourly wage. Tax deductions available through business ownership are a definite added bonus, especially with the 1987 tax laws. Private practice combined with a private business of a related nature can be a great combination.

Is seminar promoting for you? I advise you to survey what the needs and competition are in your area. Intuition is a good guide, but sound surveys of what is already out there and what dental professionals are looking for is very important. The market for a continuing education business does not remain static. Opportunities can often develop in your favor, just as they can pass out of your reach. It is important to frequent the meetings of your State Board of Dental Examiners. Their guidelines determine what courses you are allowed to issue credit for. As new members come onto the Board, ideas are changed and regulations challenged. The Boards have the power to abruptly curtail your business, so be sure to always stay abreast of contemplated rule revisions.

A business such as Health Spectrum need not be the end product. I am now placing many of my speakers at national dental meetings. This is a service valued by my speakers, as well as the associations that are always looking for speakers with superb delivery and excellent material. Planning agendas for out-of-the country dental travel seminars for other organizations is another area that utilizes my seminar planning skills. I now consider any educational enterprise with a dental emphasis to be my field of expertise.

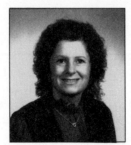

Marsha Raff

*[Interested readers can contact Marsha Raff at **Health Spectrum**, P.O. Box 356, Millbrae, CA 94030. Tel. (415) 692-5167.]*

RDH as Practice Owner

Profile of **Beverly Brill Jenkins,** *RDH, sole proprietor of* **Dental Hygiene Associates** *in Portland, Oregon.*

An energetic, enthusiastic doer, Beverly Brill Jenkins has been involved in dentistry for over 30 years and in dental hygiene for more than fifteen.

Along with her many other involvements, she operates a volunteer employment referral service for the Oregon Dental Hygienists' Association.

With the 1980 amendment in the Oregon Dental Practice Act which allows dental hygienists to practice under the general supervision of a practicing dentist, Beverly realized her long-awaited dream of establishing a sole proprietorship dental hygiene practice.

Her practice is located in a medical-dental complex in downtown Portland. She and her independent contractor/associates provide dental hygiene services in accordance with the Oregon Dental Hygiene Practice Act.

Prior to Beverly's business venture, she took courses in management, business, finance and administration. Then after months of legal and financial transactions, plus the commitment and encouragement of her former employers, she accepted the risk and responsibility of owning her own dental hygiene practice in the fall of 1980.

Start Up

To keep my capital investment within reasonable means, I searched for good previously-owned equipment.

It really paid to shop around. Through careful hunting, I was able to purchase all my needed equipment which included three treatment chairs and delivery systems, operator chairs, X-ray unit, automatic developer, instruments, cabinets, and business office equipment.

I found a dental instrument company that was going out of business. The owner sold me $5000 worth of instruments for $2500—a great savings! I also discovered better pricing at medical supply houses especially for masks, gloves and disposable paper/plastic products.

I entered into a sublease agreement and contract with a general practice dentist. This gave me full control of an adjoining office for my dental hygiene practice. The dentist provides the necessary authorization and general supervision for dental hygiene treatment and welcomes the referrals from **Dental Hygiene Associates.**

It took about six months before I began to see a return on my investment. It would have been sooner had I not been embezzled by a new employee. That was as much of a shock as it was a loss.

RDH Staff

Associated with me are two hygienists who are independent contractor/associates of the practice. They earn a fixed fifty percent of their net production. Services include routine prophylaxis, periodontal scaling and maintenance, root planing, gingival curettage, local anesthetic, fluoride treatments, bitewings, full-mouth intraoral and extraoral radiographs, soft tissue evaluation, perio probing and charting, nutritional counseling and home care instructions. Each patient receives oral physiotherapy aids at each appointment.

I also employ dental hygienists who work on a limited basis when either I or my associates are on vacation, ill, or attending a postgraduate course. Last year, there was a total of 15 RDHs on staff at various times. This eliminated canceling of previously scheduled patients.

Because mine is such a unique practice, I receive many requests from RDHs who want to work in such an environment. Someday, I hope to own a dental hygiene practice in the Carribean and offer a two-week "working vacation" for hygienists from the continental United States. Remember, "The turtle makes progress only when she sticks her neck out!"

Patient Base

Before embarking on my new career direction, I had, in my previous years as an employee, built a strong base of dental hygiene patients. My practice now includes those patients plus a considerable increase of new patients. Approximately 4,500 appointments a year are scheduled.

I also offer dental hygiene services at a fifty percent reduction in fees to other RDHs, dental assistants, dental technicians, and dentists who do not employ a hygienist. It's an eye-opener to realize that a portion of that statistical fifty percent of the population who never seek professional dental care are dental professionals! Also, *Senior Smile* and handicapped patients are offered a fifty percent fee reduction.

Benefits of Being in Business

These are some of the benefits I have received in my transition from employee to business owner:

- job security
- professional recognition
- personal growth
- respect of the community
- close association with interested peers
- control of my life and professional convictions
- positive self-image
- opportunity to provide a specialized health service
- opportunity to teach as well as learn
- opportunity to employ dental hygienists and assistants
- opportunity to exercise management and administrative skills
- opportunity to direct energies towards achieving goals
- opportunity to travel and speak about practice
- opportunity to increase income
- choice of working hours and vacations
- greater tax advantages

When you are an employee, you "take what you can get," but when you are self-employed, you "work for what you want."

Owning a dental hygiene practice is a viable alternative to employee status with or without general supervision. However, as in any business, there is the element of risk. You have to put in extremely long hours sacrificing a good income while building your practice and image. But remember the adage, "The height that great (wo)men reached and kept was not obtained by sudden flight; but they, while their companions slept, were toiling upward in the night."

How Dentists Benefit

Dentists also benefit from my practice because we:

- assume the responsibility of providing and recording all preventive procedures to patients of record and new patients
- generate restorative procedures to the dental staff
- provide preliminary caries charting and tissue evaluation
- take complete medical histories, radiographs and perioprobings
- keep dental staff informed of any changes in patient's health
- comply with all applicable federal, state, county, and city statutes, ordinances and regulations
- are solely liable for any and all expenses incurred for self and independent contractor/associates

Further the dentists:

- are not obligated to pay any sums of money whatsoever for dental hygiene services rendered to shared patients
- have no obligation to contribute to RDH's:

—overhead	—retirement
—income	—profit sharing
—continuing education	—unemployment tax
—social security	—workmen's compensation
—federal and state tax	—malpractice insurance
—uniforms and upkeep	—instruments and supplies
—med/dent insurance	—disability insurance

In short, the dental hygienist assumes the responsibility of being self-employed. And, as I've said before, "although our practices are financially independent of each other, together we provide total comprehensive oral health care."

How the Patients Gain

The benefits to the patient in our consumer-oriented culture are considerable. They include:

- greater public access to a specialized service
- the opportunity to receive a regularly scheduled dental hygiene appointment with the hygienist of their choice
- the opportunity to have an exam by a dentist the same day as RDH appointment
- well-established perio and preventive maintenance program
- dental hygiene fees are commensurate with like fees in the area
- RDH has credibility not only as a licensed professional, but as a consumer of dentistry, which can be a direct influence.

So you see, everyone benefits.

I would be happy to discuss what I am doing with any interested RDH or dental/dental hygiene groups. For further information about my speaking/consulting services, contact me at **Dental Hygiene Associates,** 216 No. Hayden Bay Drive, Portland, OR 97217-7912. Tel. 503/286-4025.

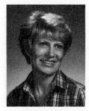

Beverley Brill Jenkins

Seven Key Points
for Career Changers

- *Take a personal accounting of yourself.* Draw a line down the center of a piece of paper. On one side list your strong points; on the other, your weaknesses. Maybe you like to work with people as part of a team but lack the discipline to see a project through on your own. Maybe your "stick-to-itiveness" or detail-sticklering would make you better suited to an administrative post than someone else. Perhaps you don't write well but are terrific speaking one-on-one or to groups.

  Include in your lists those qualities you've learned about yourself from your volunteer work. Maybe spending time at a nursing home taught you you're patient with old people. Put it down. The list will grow and from it will emerge the portrait of an individual better suited to some kinds of positions than others.

- *Give up the armchair.* You're not likely to find the right job showing up in the want ads or by waiting for someone to call you. You've got to "pound the pavement." Job hunting, with its inevitable rejections, is hard on your self-confidence. That's why it's so important to know yourself. If you downplay your abilities, you'll go after jobs for which you will be unsuited; if you overinflate your self-image, you'll spend lots of time chasing the wrong goals.

- *Decide who or what you'd like to work for or in.* Find people in similar situations and ask them what they do in their jobs, what the challenges are, the routines, the opportunities, the requirements. You may find you have a distorted or unreal idea of a particular career, especially in the so-called "glamorous" ones. (See section on Sales.)

- *Watch your résumé.* Make sure you make a clear statement of your job objective and purpose, backed up by appropriate experience.

- *Budget your resources.* Changing your career direction takes time and money: for résumé copies, postage, long-distance calls, an out-of-town trip, lunches to develop leads. At the same time you've got to meet your normal living costs. Plan your resources to cover both.

• **Don't bail out too soon.**   Before quitting one job, try to find another. It's not easy to manage a full-time job, personal life, and look for another career goal at the same time. But it can be done if you use vacation and after-hours time. Sticking with the old job will take the financial pressure off while you're looking. Changes take time: yours.

• **Use personal contacts.**   Whether they're professional colleagues, acquaintances, relatives, favorite educators, friends, whatever, tell them you're "looking." True, you won't get a job just by using "pull," but your contacts can open doors. What happens then is up to you.

*An excellent resource for evaluating your personal interests and professional opportunities is *"Contracting for Services in Alternative Practice Settings."*

This self-study course authored by Beverly Entwistle, RDH, MPH and Bonnie Bruerd, RDH, MPH is available through the Division of Professional Development, ADHA, 444 No. Mich. Ave., Suite 3400, Chicago, IL 60611. Tel. 312/440-8900.

RDH in Industry

RDH in Industrial Research

Elaine Satin *turns an academic interest in microbiology into an income-producing career in research.*

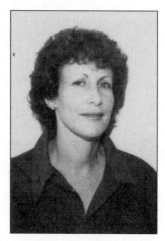

Elaine Satin

Pursuing An Interest

My own evolution into dental research began rather unintentionally while I was in dental hygiene school. I enjoyed microbiology and decided to take some advanced courses in that area. To my surprise, I was told that these courses were not available to dental hygiene students. I recall thinking how rigid our curriculum was. Nevertheless, my interest in microbiology remained, and I kept the interest alive to some degree by reading dental research journals. This is a habit that I am very glad that I developed; dental journals and some trade magazines are the main sources of information on contemporary research. Even if you have only a superficial understanding of research findings and methods, this knowledge is an important foundation that can be built upon whenever you need to do so.

When I went on for my bachelor's degree, I took several liberal arts courses that required research papers. Although most of those courses were in the field of literature, I learned how to use the library, to critique the literature, and most importantly, how to write. This is another skill that is essential in preparing oneself for a research position.

After graduating, I worked in private practice for about four years. Throughout this period I began to feel out of touch with my education. I had learned so much, yet I used so little of it on the job. I knew that I needed a more stimulating work situation. I wasn't sure what I wanted to do, I just knew that it had to be different from what I was doing.

A community college near my town had recently begun a two-year dental hygiene program. I sent in an application to teach, had an interview, and was accepted as an instructor. I needed a master's degree in dental hygiene, so I began graduate school at the same time that I began teaching.

In graduate school, I found that research studies were often in progress in various departments within the dental school. I asked some of my dental hygiene and dental student classmates about the studies. Many of their remarks were erroneous and/or negative, i.e. "it's boring; why would you want to do that; you have to have a Ph.D. or a D.D.S. to really get involved," etc. Fortunately, I met a dental hygienist in one of my classes who had some positive comments to make as she had been a research assistant in the preventive dentistry department.

I made an appointment with the director of the preventive dentistry department. He was very encouraging. He said that if I had the interest and the ability to learn, then I could be trained to become a research assistant. The fact that I was teaching and going to graduate school and therefore had at best, about six hours available, did not appear to be a drawback. He and his research staff would train me and if I proved to be reliable and patient, I could learn a great deal about dental research. My salary would be minimal; I would be paid when and if money from research grants became available. My feeling about this last point is that I was being trained by one of the top dental researchers in the world. I felt fortunate to be in this situation, therefore, money was certainly not an issue. Anyone who makes money an issue is missing the point; it will come later. Pay your dues first.

This was the key experience that gave me the opportunity to decide if research was what I wanted. I participated in several different studies, usually as a technician, although I occasionally got involved in the organizational aspects of the study such as protocol development, subject recruitment, and scheduling. I was aware of the industry representatives meeting with the university researchers to discuss the type of study that they (from industry) wanted to place. In time, I was able to directly or indirectly participate in the whole process of conducting a study. It does take time to figure out who does what, when and why.

Learning As You Go

I kept a journal of my experiences, recording the studies that I participated in, the products being tested, test sponsors, and materials and methods used. I read as much as I could about the product(s) and the objective(s). For example, if we were testing the ability of mouthwash A to more effectively inhibit mouth odor than mouthwash B or C, I would read about how mouthwash inhibits odors, which ingredients are most effective in accomplishing this, and how other studies have been designed to test this hypothesis. It made me feel more confident, and I was better able to converse with my colleagues about our rationale for designing the study a particular way. I also checked ingredients on over-the-counter dental products. What is the difference between *Lavoris, Listerine* and *Scope?* Is it simply the taste, or is one really more effective than the other? And why? I took an interest in what I was doing. My colleagues noticed, and I was given more responsibility.

I was now asked to review protocols and I was "let in" on some of the conversations between industry and the research group. I don't teach in the summer so I was able to devote more time to research. I was taught how to collect, weigh, and store plaque samples, measure sulcular fluid, and operate a pH meter. I began my own personal research file, photocopying articles that pertained to any of the studies with which I had been involved. I became a member of the International Association of Dental Research and subscribed to several research journals. Finally, upon completing a plaque pH study, I wrote and published an article.

Taking Stock

I now had my master's degree in dental hygiene, one and a half years as a research assistant, four years of teaching dental hygiene, and was pregnant with my first child. I knew I had to cut down on my schedule so I made the decision to leave my research position. I felt reasonably certain that I could re-enter the research field at the right time.

When my son was five months old I returned to teaching. I found that my research training had a positive effect on my teaching. I was not as willing to accept "textbook theories" about the science and practice of dental hygiene.

For instance, in clinic I had always encouraged the students to polish the teeth thoroughly after a scaling. Then, I read some literature about selective polishing and an evaluation of the whole issue of when, if, and how often to polish. I showed the articles to the students and we discussed the topic thoroughly; everyone agreed that we should adopt this practice in our clinic. We began to (re)educate our patients as well as our colleagues.

I invited two dental hygienists who had published an article on this subject to speak to the class. Research had prompted me to investigate this and many other areas, and I believe it has had a favorable impact on my students.

Into Consulting

Two years after I left my research assistant job, I received a call from a research dentist who I had met at a dental materials symposium. At this point I'd like to impress upon you how vital it is to keep in touch with the people you meet in the field. An occasional phone call or note is all that is necessary to keep you in their minds. Anyway, this person was working as a dental consultant for an independent laboratory requiring someone with my background to help develop their dental area. I went for the interview and was notified that the position of dental hygiene consultant was mine.

The independent laboratory generally provides the same type of testing services as does the university. In fact, they compete with each other for studies from industry. This laboratory was well established in the medical and pharmaceutical area and now wished to expand their services to include dentistry. Since my teaching schedule prevented me from being available for clinical studies (these studies usually require three to five days per week participation), I would concentrate on protocol review and development for clients, and I would meet with clients to explain our services.

I was given a mini-course in the types of testing conducted by the laboratory. The laboratory tests cosmetics, drugs, and household products for their safety and efficacy. These two types of studies are very different in their design and their objectives. Safety studies seek to find out if products are safe for human use. Side effects such as skin irritation and allergic reactions have to be closely monitored. Efficacy studies have to do with advertising claims such as Brand A toothbrush removes plaque more thoroughly than Brand B toothbrush. Often the Food and Drug Administration (FDA) will challenge a company to provide more clinical evidence in their support of a claim.

I have learned a great deal about federal rules and regulations governing studies. This includes the FDA as well as other governmental health agencies, and the Institutional Review Board, a group of professionals who review study proposals and decide if the study is safe and ethical. I have also become familiar with various laws and agen-

135

cies (such as the Environmental Protection Agency) that have been established to protect the public from toxic wastes, environmental pollution, and testing of unknown substances on confined groups of people, such as prisoners (no longer allowed). Panelists who volunteer to participate in studies must sign an informed consent form. This form states what the panelist is to do, any risks involved, who to contact if there is any adverse reaction, and panelist exclusions (minors, pregnant women, individuals with systemic illnesses, etc.).

I have now been a consultant for three and a half years. This position has expanded upon my former position in university research. While I am able to work in a technical capacity in studies during the summer months, I am mostly involved in client communications. I concentrate on contracting studies from industry. I meet with the research and development divisions of major corporations. I present our capabilities; they describe their needs. If they are interested in placing their study with us, we write a cost estimate. Companies "shop around" for the best price, just as consumers do.

Just as there is excitement when a study is contracted, there is great disappointment when a company retracts a study at the last minute. Sometimes a lot of preparation has been made in anticipation of a study: a protocol has been developed, a panel has been assembled, a group of technicians have been scheduled. Then the company decides to work with a university or their marketing group has decided to re-evaluate the product. You must learn to expect these defeats. Nothing is certain until a contract has been signed.

Right now, for my particular life style and with a second child, I find that five to seven hours per week is about as much as I can devote to my consulting position. My manager does not pressure me into working more hours; additional staff members absorb any extra hours. There is a minimal amount of travel; usually a few clients may be located about 100 miles away. There are also three or four research meetings per year, although most of them are local. The salary is quite good, and an expense account is available if you require it.

When my children are older I may be able to accept a larger role in the company. I also feel that there are other research options available to me.

In conclusion, I feel that my dental hygiene education served as a good foundation in my path to research. If you are thinking about a research career, I would suggest that you take courses in research writing, communications, and business (specifically marketing). Look for an apprenticeship in university research much like what I described earlier. Be flexible in your thinking, and above all, be patient.

RDH in Dental Product Sales

Shelley Sullivan *moved out of the private practice environment into representing the products of a dental manufacturer.*

After attending my first national dental convention as a dental hygiene student, I knew what I wanted to do with my career.

Every February the dental hygiene class would make a trip to the Chicago Midwinter Dental Meeting to attend lectures the ADHA sponsored and to view the exhibits. It was there that I met many hygienists who had used dental hygiene as a steppingstone to become dentists, business consultants, researchers, and professional salespeople.

These women seemed very sophisticated, well-educated, well-groomed and independent to me. I was captivated. After meeting and speaking with some of them, I was encouraged to pursue a bachelor's degree in business along with dental hygiene. This I did.

After Graduation

When I completed my education, I found employment in a very unusual dental office in Chicago. The dentist/employer was a Greek national who spoke seven languages fluently. In addition to regular Greek patients, my office served two local janitorial unions. Here I met people from Yugoslavia, Romania and The Soviet Union who spoke little or no English. Many of them exhibited poor dental health.

I was quite challenged by the situation. I learned a great deal about oral pathology, deep scaling and curettage, and how to deal with the language barrier. How do you effectively teach preventive care to patients who had never seen a toothbrush before, never mind a dentist!

But after two years of this, my interest began to wane. My salary had leveled off and benefits were non-existent. No matter how hard I worked, or how much business I brought to the practice, my efforts went unrewarded. I also didn't like the fact that my income was dependent on the dentist's presence in the office. There were many vacations, sick days, and "I don't feel like working" days I had to contend with.

Taking the Plunge

Remembering those RDHs I had met and admired, I rewrote my résumé to capitalize on the fact that I *sold* dentistry to my patients as well as promote many preventive products for home care. I was going for a position in sales.

137

I put on my best "serious" suit. I was the first to arrive when the next Chicago dental convention opened. Nervously clutching my résumé, I passed it out to anyone who would take it.

The meeting proved to be a gold mine of resources. Here under one roof were managers and executives of dental companies nationwide. I landed *five* interviews!

I accepted a position as a laboratory salesperson, promoting certified lab technologies to area dentists in the St. Louis market.

The company provided me with a car, health and life insurance, an expense account and paid for my move to a new city. I was sent to a professional sales training course to sharpen my selling skills.

Financially, though, I didn't come out ahead. I had to take a cut in pay because of my lack of sales experience. And, although I had many selling successes, I became dissatisfied with my straight salary and no commissions on my sales. My motivation dropped off.

Incredibly, it was at this point that a sales manager from a dental manufacturer contacted me for an opening in the Ohio, Indiana, West Virginia market. He had kept my year-old résumé from that important (for me) Chicago meeting! I jumped at the opportunity.

Unfortunately, nine months after I was hired, the company went out of business and I was out of a job.

A "head hunter" contacted me and I obtained a position with another dental manufacturer. This meant yet another relocation, now to the Michigan area where I am currently working.

What I Do

As a dental materials representative for a wholesale manufacturer of dental products and equipment, my function is to increase and promote the sale and use of my company's products in my assigned geographical territory.

To accomplish this, I serve as a combination educator, troubleshooter and resource person for dental supply houses, schools with dental programs, and government providers of dental care.

My customers are mainly the supply houses who employ representatives to service dentists, the end users of my products. I am known in the industry as a "manufacturer's rep."

My job involves many areas of sales and promotion. I make weekly and monthly calls to 15 supply houses in Michigan and Ohio. During these calls, I check inventory, return credits or damaged merchandise, leave literature for the reps, and educate the inside workers and the managers on my product line. My goal is to help suppliers move my company's merchandise off their shelves and encourage them to buy on a continual basis.

I try to make myself as visible as possible by scheduling sales meetings and co-traveling with the 148 supply house representatives in my territory.

Co-traveling means riding with each rep for a day at a time, making sales presentations to their dentist/accounts to educate them on my products. The objective is to have the rep promote my products over my competitor's.

It can be tough. Not only do you have to try to sell each doctor in a very limited amount of time, you must be able to adapt and relate to 148 different personalities.

I also work at various national dental trade shows. I enjoy traveling, but many times the only thing I ever see is the convention hall and the airport!

Pros and Cons of the Job

I must say I love what I do. It is very rewarding to me to be able to give advice, discuss technique and sell a dentist on the benefits of my products. However, the job can be lonely and one must become very resourceful when traveling alone, especially when you have a flat tire in the middle of nowhere!

I am presently single so the job fits my career goals and life style. But if I were married and raising a family—which I hope to do some day—private practice would be a perfect alternative to sales for me.

Salaries and Benefits

Requirements for the job vary, but usually a degree and sales experience are necessary. Starting salaries can range from $20,000 to $27,000 depending on ability, experience and education.

On top of that, monthly commissions or quarterly bonuses are paid on the amount of sales generated in your territory. This creates a high motivation. You can determine your income. The potential is unlimited.

Included in my non-taxable fringe benefits are full medical and dental coverage, paid vacation and sick leave, retirement, disability and life insurance plans, a company car and an expense account for business travel and entertainment. I work out of my home and have a tremendous amount of freedom and flexibility in scheduling myself.

Tips on Getting a Sales Position

My advice is to be a master at what you are doing *now*. Be the best clinical hygienist you can be, learn about the products in your practice, assist the doctor and staff, be invaluable as an employee. Then when you are ready to move on, you'll feel confident of your abilities.

Contact your local supply house rep and discuss your interest in sales. He or she can show you trade publications that advertise sales positions and can put you in touch with the various wholesale representatives in the area. Try to take some sales courses or get selling experience even if it is not dentally related.

Be sure to attend local and national dental trade shows with your résumé. Look what it did for me!

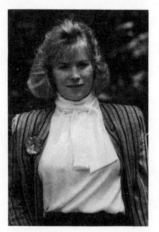

Shelley Sullivan

*[Interested readers can contact Shelley Sullivan through **Career Directions for Dental Hygienists**.]*

RDH in Marketing

Denise Sabol *has transferred her skills and knowledge to marketing professional products for a dental manufacturer.*

Leaving a top rung on one career ladder to begin at the bottom rung of another was a choice I had no idea of making as I entered the work force of dental hygiene professionals. Just out of dental hygiene school, I felt committed to my career choice and anxious to discover the real world of private practice.

Since that time, fourteen years ago, I have worked in various private practice settings and enjoyed seven years of teaching dental hygiene. I've been satisfied with my career in dental hygiene (sometimes more, sometimes less), and have always felt a commitment or attachment to it.

In striving to fulfill my personal and professional goals, I decided to pursue a career move into the dental products industry, expanding into a new area while building upon my experiences in dental hygiene. I have succeeded in transferring my skills into marketing and am an assistant product manager for a dental products manufacturing company.

The changes along my career path have often been spurned by feelings of restlessness, emptiness, and sometimes boredom, culminating in a desire to discover and learn something new. At each point of decision I asked myself, "Should I change practice settings?" "Should I get my degree?" "Should I try teaching?" I struggled with the disturbing feelings of indecision. My most difficult career move was choosing to leave a full-time dental hygiene teaching position and transfer my skills to the dental products industry.

After Teaching—What?

I had experienced a lot of anxiety over the thought of leaving the familiar, comfortable job expectations of teaching. Seven years of teaching dental hygiene had bred a lot of familiarity and friendship. I wrestled with the conflict of comfort versus challenge for nearly two years before making my decision to act.

My hesitancy was broken when I realized I did not see myself teaching for the rest of my life; or the next ten years; or the next five! I sincerely enjoyed teaching but needed to start a new learning/discovery curve based on my knowledge of dental hygiene, teaching . . . and myself. Teaching was something to return to. Now it was time to leave.

I had grown competent and confident in my field of work, owning a strong positive attitude about myself and my capabilities. This self-resolution was essential in making my decision to leave "traditional dental hygiene," and helped me tremendously throughout my job hunt and beyond.

Once I decided to leave teaching and explore other avenues, I experienced a sense of freedom in having made my decision, and was motivated by the excitement of the challenge and risk involved.

Returning to private practice as a means of financial support, I began a one and a half year "job" of exploring, self-assessment, and career redirection.

Action Plan

Reading books and attending classes on skills assessment, career planning, résumé writing, and networking sounds pretty dry but was an active way to begin my self-assessment.

For the first time, I was writing a résumé targeting a field outside of dental hygiene. How should I begin? How would I convince a stranger in an unrelated field of work I am capable and qualified?

I had never before had to "hunt" for a job, and the experience was lonely, discouraging, difficult and frustrating. There were no shortcuts to this job search campaign. What did I want to do? Where did I want to do it? How was I going to get there? These questions were short enough but the answers necessitated some lengthy processes of research, self-assessment, and goal setting.

Through these career and life planning exercises[1] I was able to define my most marketable skills and target my career goals into three areas: marketing, sales, and training. I tailored a résumé to suit each of these job objectives. I answered newspaper ads, contacted people I knew in my targeted, or related, fields of work, conducted information-gathering interviews, and completed library research on companies before making application to a job and/or before interviews.

I also utilized any contacts I was able to make chairside, after developing a rapport with patients in the course of my normal work day in private practice. The "patient resources" that visited my operatory were supportive and helpful. Of course, using patients as resources depends on the relationship you have with the dentist you work with and whether you have shared your goals with him/her. However, you can always finish your discussions with your "patient resources" on the phone after work hours.

[1] Bolles, Richard Nelson. *What Color Is Your Parachute?: A Practical Manual for Job-Hunters and Career Changes.* Ten Speed Press, Berkeley, California. 1980. (Editions revised annually).

As I pursued various avenues in my job search, I was able to further define my goals experiencing several job interviews, rejecting a few offers and being rejected. It was becoming clear to me that my interests were in discovering more about marketing.

Finally, through a combination of resources, i.e. newspaper, friends, professional contacts, I was offered, and accepted, a position in marketing as assistant product manager for a dental products manufacturing company. Although an M.B.A. is normally required for this entry-level position in marketing, the cards happened to be in my favor weighing my experience in the dental field, master's degree in technical education, and the particular job opening.

Well, this was it. I had substituted my curets and prophy angles for pencils and a calculator. It did not take long to discover that the business of marketing was the business of producing a *product* to match the needs of a consumer—and make money from it; while the business of dentistry and dental hygiene was the business of providing a *service* to match the needs of a patient—and make a profit.

Instead of sitting chairside scaling, I was sitting at a desk calculating numbers generating financial data. The task of organizing dental office inventory and managing money for supplies was converted to managing advertising and sales budgets, and forecasting sales.

Transferring Skills

The rapport I maintained with every patient and the members of the dental office team was the same type of communication necessary to get things done in the much larger environment of a company and its many departments.

Just as I had kept current on state legislation and ADHA curriculum guidelines, I have followed up on Food and Drug Administration regulations and American Dental Association certification guidelines as they affect products I manage.

The initiative and creativity needed to develop outlines, objectives and course materials was the same stuff needed to develop strategies and objectives for selling aids, marketing plans or packaging changes.

The experience gained in speaking before people, i.e. chairside, lecturing, community groups, has proven to be invaluable when making presentations of business propositions, marketing plans, or at sales meetings.

Above all, the perseverence, patience, stamina and commitment used in everyday private practice and teaching have been the most valuable skills transferred to a field unrelated, one might assume, to dental hygiene.

Pros and Cons

My transition onto a new career ladder has invited opportunity and sacrifices. The trade-off for challenge and a better salary has been longer work hours, less time for personal life, and a higher stress level.

The most notable aspect of transferring from traditional dental hygiene into marketing has been the acute challenge presented to my own sense of confidence and competency. Beneath the anxiety and stress that change brings, I have carried a strong determination to reach my next goal and discover my capabilities. My transition into marketing has given me a greater level of personal satisfaction knowing I have achieved my goal.

The hierarchical structure of marketing offers opportunities for advancement for those who seek to climb the career ladder. Job titles may vary from one company to another (managers versus directors) but product management has a ranked order allowing for promotion from assistant manager to manager to senior manager to group manager, etc. The salary range for entry level positions is found in the low twenties to low thirties depending on experience.

Should my priorities shift in the future, I may consider returning to private practice or teaching. I have come to realize that the self-evaluation process to establish and prioritize my personal and professional goals must be, at the very least, a frequent one.

It takes a well-thought-out self-assessment followed by a targeted goal and commitment to it, to obtain the type of job you want. Goal setting and believing in yourself is extremely important. It is equally important to reassess your goals and yourself based on what you've learned along the way.

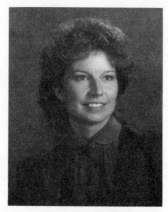

Denise Sabol

RDH
Working Abroad

A Guide To Working Abroad

Claudine Paula Drew *explains step-by-step how to work abroad recounting both her own experience and those of her colleagues.*

You've thought and thought about it. You know that others have done it, so why not you? You love to travel, seek new adventures and conquer new situations. In fact, you need an exciting challenge. Why not do it? Why *not* work in a foreign country?

I have always been a curious person, especially when it comes to knowing how other people in other lands live their lives. Are we more alike than different in our values, hopes, wishes and loves? What better way to find out than first hand. I made a commitment to myself that I would live and work overseas for one year.

Where To Begin

My first step was to make sure that my passport was up-to-date and in order. A passport is a formal document issued by the government to its citizens. It officially establishes the bearer's identity and nationality, and authorizes the bearer to travel outside his/her own country.

To get the necessary information and application, I called the Hall of Records located in the courthouse of the county in which I live. Some states permit applications to be issued through the post office. Ask your postal clerk. Another alternative is to contact the Passport Field Agency nearest you at the following zip codes: Boston 02203, Chicago 60604, Detroit 48226, Honolulu 96850, Houston 77002, Los Angeles 90261, Miami 33130, New Orleans 70130, New York 10021, Philadelphia 19106, San Francisco 94102, Seattle 98174, Stamford, CT 06901, and Washington, D.C. 20524. These agencies also have publications you can request. Two that might prove helpful are "You and Your Passport" and "Visa Requirements of Foreign Governments." (More on visas coming up.)

The clerk at the Hall of Records told me what to do. I had to physically present myself to them bringing my birth certificate to prove I was born in the United States and/or the child of American citizens. Also, I was to bring two identical photographs in either color or black and white. One was for the passport application, the other for the actual

146

passport. I did this and was assured I would receive my passport in six to eight weeks. It would be valid for ten years from the date of issuance. My first step was now completed.

About Visas

Many countries require a visa for entrance. A visa is an endorsement placed or stamped in the passport by a counsular or embassy official of the foreign country. It indicates that the passport document has been examined and the bearer has complied with the requirements for entry. The visa allows that bearer to travel within the foreign country.

There are two types of visas: a temporary or tourism visa, and a working visa or permit. The tourism visa is good for only a short period of time, usually two to six months; the working visa, for a period of one to two years. To obtain the working visa, you need proof of employment. Your new employer/dentist will assist you in your visa requirements. He then becomes your sponsor.

Obtain a copy of the latest edition of Visa Requirements of Foreign Governments, published by the State Department Bureau of Consular Affairs. This document is for sale by the Superintendent of Documents, U.S. Government Printing Office, Washington, D.C. 20402. It may also be found at some post offices.

Which Country to Work In?

My second step was to choose specifically *which* challenging, new, foreign land. Did I want Australia? Hong Kong? Switzerland? England? Saudi Arabia? Or even next door, Canada? I was not too sure. I decided to investigate what was available.

I wrote to the ADHA, 444 N. Michigan Avenue, Suite 3400, Chicago, IL 60611 requesting their list, "Foreign Employment—Information and Referrals". This list includes the countries of Australia, Africa, Canada, England, Germany, Holland, Japan, Norway, Sweden and Switzerland, among others. It even includes the addresses of organizations such as Project Hope, Pan American Health Organization and The Salvation Army.

Another useful resource for names and addresses is the booklet, "National and International Dental Organizations of the World." Send a $5 check to the Council on International Relations, ADA, 211 East Chicago Avenue, Chicago, IL 60611. With this booklet, you will have the addresses of dental agencies in other countries. You can then write to each one in which you are interested requesting information on employment and possible employers.

147

A third approach—one which I used—was to call the embassy of the foreign country in which I was interested. Embassies and consulates are located in all major cities. If you can't locate them through your telephone book, ask your local public librarian in which directory you would find their addresses.

I researched the possibility of working in Australia. The Australian Embassy was most helpful. (It certainly is a delight to hear the different accents. Most countries import their own citizens to work in their embassies.) They sent me an application for a working permit and gave me addresses of dental agencies to contact in Australia.

Another embassy I had contacted (of Saudi Arabia), although non-commital, did suggest I write to the Ministry of Health, Riyadh, Saudi Arabia. My request was soon returned to me from the Ministry stating they did not hire hygienists.

Classified ads in professional journals are another resource for you to consider. In such sections within our own ADHA journal I have often found foreign dentists seeking American hygienists. In fact, a few years ago, I answered an ad from a dentist in Milano, Italy. I had a delightful correspondence with him for the next four months. He even wrote to me in Saudi Arabia (where I ended up) to wish me well!

Reverse this procedure. If potential employers can advertise for us in our journal, then why can't we, potential employees, advertise for foreign dentists in the ADA journal? The Journal of the American Dental Association is widely read throughout the world. Pick your country, include your address, and tell them you have curet, will travel!

Also, if you have friends living in that foreign land you've picked, ask them to place a "Position Wanted" ad in the local newspaper. They can have it translated into the appropriate language, and who knows, you just might find your prospective employer that way.

My last suggestion is to network among friends. Those friends (including dentists), who travel extensively, may know of dentists in other countries. In fact, there is a dentist in New York City who is active in placing volunteer dental personnel on a kibbutz in Israel. For more information write American Volunteers for Israel, 108-13 67th Rd., Forest Hills, NY 11375. Bear in mind that volunteering is a good way to go over and stay for a month or so to see if you like the country well enough to live there for a longer time.

On Making Choices

I knew my commitment was to work abroad, but I still didn't know where. I had done some traveling in 1981 and found myself in Hong Kong, a city with which I fell in love. I took a day off from the tour and taxied up to the University of Hong Kong. I introduced myself to the recruitment office and had my name and application put on file in case a position became available.

Then I took a taxi to the American Embassy. I introduced myself to some of the American personnel and asked who their dentist was in Hong Kong, and did he or she have a hygienist. Sure enough, one did. An American!

Off I went for the third time that day. (I saw a lot of Hong Kong even without the tour!) This hygienist said she would keep me in mind if any post opened up. To date, she is still there—but one never knows! (I must interject that I met so many nice people who were most anxious to help. The same will be true for you.)

It is a good idea to visit the country before you move there. That is why volunteering can be a boost. Of course, it is not always possible. It wasn't in my case. My final choice was the Kingdom of Saudi Arabia. There is no tourism in Saudi Arabia because the Moslems feel that the country must be kept holy for the Moslem pilgrims who travel to Mecca for the holy days of Haj. These pilgrims come from all over the world. Consequently, the Saudi Arabian government issues only working visas.

However, if you do visit a country that captures your fancy while vacationing, why not investigate your working options? Check the American Embassy for information, check the local dental societies for prospective employers, put an ad in the local paper giving your U.S.A. address for response, try to find if there is a dental hygienists association, ask the hotel where you are staying which dentist they recommend for guests who have a toothache. Then call that doctor to ask if he can be of assistance to you in your quest for a job.

My final choice, as I said, was the Kingdom of Saudi Arabia. Why? Because I knew of no one who had worked there and because I knew very little about the country itself. A completely new adventure! I secured my job through a hiring agency for the King Faisal Specialist Hospital and Research Hospital in Riyadh, Saudi Arabia (sounds exotic, doesn't it? It was!)

I had tried a few leads prior to my appointment, first through Aramco Services Company, Foreign Services Employment Department, 1100 Milam, Houston, TX 77002. We exchanged a few phone calls over a period of ten months, but nothing materialized. Most of my leads for this country came through my networking among my friends and colleagues.

In all, it took me eighteen months to actually find employment. This is not an unusual time span for this particular country. I was eventually hired by the Hospital Corporation of America, International Division, One Park Plaza, P.O. Box 550, Nashville, TN 37202. They assisted me in obtaining a working visa from the Government of Saudi Arabia. There was much paperwork to be taken care of, but remember, the sponsoring employer will help you.

Necessary Credentials

First, I had to present proof of graduation from an accredited dental hygiene school. I photocopied my degrees. This was sufficient. You will find that the United States has the best training programs for any professional. (Excuse me while I wave the flag. One of the advantages of living overseas is that you do come to appreciate the U.S. even more.) The licenses and registrations for professional degrees will more than satisfy foreign employers. No advanced courses will be needed except if you want to take a language course for that foreign country in which you will soon be living.

Recommendations from present employers, from your dental hygiene instructors, from your clergyman, and character references from friends will be needed. I even had to have the local police department verify that I was not wanted for any crimes!

Working experience here in the States should consist of at least two years or even three before you venture overseas. In Saudi Arabia very few Americans were hired under the age of twenty-five. This is not necessarily true for other countries.

Snapshots (passport size) will be needed for the different paperwork. I needed about a dozen black and white ones. Also, include your résumé. A physical examination might be required.

There is sometimes a lot of footwork involved in securing the necessary documents, but nothing you can't handle. Just make a list of everything needed, give yourself time to accomplish it, and start checking off the completed items. Before you know it, you will be granted that working visa through the U.S.-located embassy or consulate of the foreign country.

Other Countries, Other Requirements

Working in Switzerland, a favorite of many RDHs, calls for a completely different approach. You can file your papers with a central placement service. When a hygiene post becomes available, you will be notified. It would be best to have a sponsoring dentist/employer, but if you have no leads, why not try the placement service? Write to Ms. Rosalie Kaspar, Employment Chairperson for Foreign Hygienists-Switzerland, Dental Hygiene Schule, Minervastrasse 99, 8032 Zurich, Switzerland.

However, according to Sherry Gateman, a friend who practiced in Zurich from 1982 to 1983, there are not as many job openings as there used to be because there are now more Swiss hygienists. She was lucky in securing a post there as she started her search only three months before she was hired to work beginning three months later. Her sponsoring dentist paid for her round-trip flight from New York based on her promise to stay at least one year. This is the case with most job offers. You will be provided with a round-trip ticket with your one or two-year contract.

Housing Arrangements

Along with the work commitment and round-trip airfare, housing is usually provided either free or for a nominal amount. With my employment in Saudi Arabia, housing was included in my contract. I lived in a comfortable compound. My only expenses were long-distance telephone calls and food, which was three times more expensive than in America.

Sherry Gateman was provided a Swiss apartment for a modest rent. In Australia, a sponsoring dentist would either provide you with an apartment or assist you in finding one. In England, the same would hold true. (A note here about English employment. There is a waiting list dating back to 1979 of interested American RDHs. Unemployment is very high for nationals in England so don't count on too much.) In Hong Kong, don't take the position unless an apartment is provided. Rent for an average apartment can be as high as US$2,000 to $5,000 a month!

Salaries and Taxes

Salaries are usually paid in the currency of the country. With the U.S. dollar up, you will lose money when you convert the foreign currency into U.S. dollars. Of all the countries I investigated, Saudi Arabia probably paid the highest for a clinical dental hygienist, running US$27,000 to $28,000 per year.

Switzerland pays about US$22,000 annually. Other countries range from US$18,000 to $24,000.

Check the cost of living, travel costs for your excursions, and the local income tax (if any) that must be paid to that government. Most countries do have an income tax for their "guest workers," aliens, or, as we were called in Saudi, expatriates.

There are taxes to be paid in Switzerland, England, Italy, but none in Saudi Arabia. (They have enough from their oil!) Most jobs pay

151

enough for you to live comfortably, plus give you some extra change for your excursions into other parts of the world.

The United States will expect you to file a U.S. tax form even though you have worked out of the country for that year. If you stay in a foreign land for 330 days out of 365 and make under $75,000, you will not have to pay any U.S. income tax, but you have to file the form anyway. Your accountant or the local IRS office will assist you with this. Or, you can get IRS publication #54, "Tax Guide for the U.S. Citizen Abroad." I found assistance at the U.S. embassy in Riyadh. Around April 15th, American accountants were there to assist the "expatriates" with their U.S. tax forms.

It is a good idea to register with the American Embassy once you arrive in your new country. This can be done with passport in hand and a visit to them. If disaster strikes, or a war breaks out, they know that their citizens (you) are there and will help you in returning home. (Also, embassies have the best parties and are good contacts for meeting other Americans. Great Fourth of July gatherings!)

Advantages and Disadvantages

Well, if you followed the steps, you now have a passport, chosen the country in which you wish to work, filled out all the necessary papers for the working visa, and have even secured a sponsoring employer. You are now ready to experience what living abroad is all about. There are many things to look for in this new experience; many advantages and, like all things, some disadvantages. You have to be the judge of which list is longer, but most people, including myself, feel that the good things far outweigh the negatives.

When I asked friend, Gunda Brakas, the outcome of her two-year stay in Morocco, she sighed longingly and said her horizons had been broadened immeasurably. She felt she would never be the same because doors had been opened that could never again be closed.

Gunda's experience allowed her to view what life was like in the Middle East, a view she would not have seen or known without this unique working experience.

Another friend, Judy Iovan, a secretary at the King Faisal Specialist Hospital in Riyadh, also felt that the advantages overpowered the disadvantages. Because of the tax-free situation and the paid-for living conditions, Judy is able to save many thousands of dollars a year while enjoying the international flavor that comes with overseas employment.

The major negative for Judy is the 8,000 mile spread between her and her family and friends. Judy sorely misses her loved ones, but has found new friends away from home. She is living in another culture, experiencing different values. That is something she never would have known if she had remained an employee in the U.S.A.

Sherry Gateman loved working in Zurich. At first she was concerned because she knew no Americans. But then came the monthly dental hygiene meeting in that city. There she met sixty RDHs, many of them Americans. New friends in a foreign land!

Sherry had mixed feelings about returning home as the experience had been so exhilarating. The travel part was best since Switzerland is so close to many Western European countries: Holland, Germany, Italy.

As I, Sherry had a hard time readjusting to the American life style. It took me almost eight or nine months before I could get back in the groove of working and living in the U.S. Reverse culture shock!

Living abroad is so full—the accessibility for travel, the comradeship established with new friends. It's hard to leave. With the cost of living and the tax situation here in the States, it is quite difficult on a hygienist's salary to travel as extensively.

I truly miss my unique experiences in Saudi Arabia. I miss the trips to Jordan for six days, the trips to Athens and the Greek Islands for eight days, the weekend trips to Bahrain and stopovers to London. I especially miss the lovely friends I made, including the evenings spent visiting my Arab patients' homes. What a marvelous sharing between different people! I have many fond memories of the gracious Arabian women inviting me for dinner or tea.

Another disadvantage to consider is the language barrier. Some places will have interpreters; others will expect you to learn the language during your stay. The worst that can happen is you will become bilingual. Not such a big disadvantage!

Getting to Know Yourself Better

The biggest single plus of living overseas is the opportunity it affords you for personal growth. You will find that you have to rely on yourself much more than usual. You will not have your support system, the one that buoys you up through trials and discouraging times. In becoming self-sufficient, you will have no choice but to grow. There will be good days, there will be bad days. But there will never be any better days.

So you see, you have been listening to a very satisfied dental hygienist. I was able to view life from another perspective. I was able to live life a little through someone else's eyes. I knew my dental hygiene skills before I left. Dental hygiene is dental hygiene no matter where it is practiced. But I did not know myself as well as I do now.

Bon voyage and happy growth!

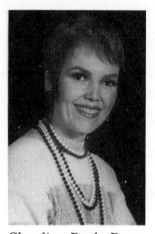

Claudine Paula Drew

*[Interested readers can contact Claudine Paula Drew through **Career Directions for Dental Hygienists.**]*

RDH in
Private Practice

RDH and the Special Patient

Mary Jean Laboissonniere *describes how her practice specialty came to be.*

I spent the first four years after graduating from hygiene school with my bachelor's degree working in private practice. However, I always scanned the ads to see if anything new was surfacing. Well, I saw an ad in the local paper for a public health hygienist.

Without having any particular training or experience in public health other than through courses in school, I applied for the position and got it! To be honest, I didn't have too much competition. There was really no one more qualified than myself to compete against.

It was a position with a regional health department which covered ten towns. I worked primarily with the school children developing a curriculum for dental health education and implementing a fluoride mouthrinse program in the schools. And, during the summer months, I had a little mobile van in which I would go around to do prophys on children.

Part of my job was to secure funds from the ten towns for the program. I had to do a lot of speaking before Boards of Education to convince them that such a program was worthwhile. Eventually, I was successful in getting the towns to contribute to the Health Department to support the program.

Developing New Skills

Doing this certainly taught me a great deal about public relations and organization. The coordination that was involved on a day-to-day basis with 15 different schools, plus my in-service work with parents called for heightening these skills.

For example, one of the problems I encountered was initial resistance from some of the teachers! They resented me coming in and taking 45 minutes of class time to do a presentation and then coming in for five minutes every week for the fluoride rinse. However, once they saw it wasn't as time-consuming as they had anticipated, got over the newness of it, and came to understand the benefits, what I was doing was accepted.

I learned that once people realize that other communities are doing a similar project with favorable results and can see the value for their community, problems disappear. Communication and time proved to be my answers.

Moving On

Since I was the only hygienist in a ten-town area, I was asked to do a lot of different things apart from the school program. I became involved with the geriatric nurse practitioner and began working with senior citizens. I was also asked to work, on a part-time basis, at a small institution for the profoundly and severely retarded.

I found that work extremely difficult at first because I had had no training in working with the handicapped. Fortunately, the consultant was a pedodontist who helped me. Eventually, I got to the point where I started to enjoy the work.

As a result of this job, I was contacted by the chief of dental public health for the state of Rhode Island. I knew him both through school and through the hygiene association in which I had been quite active. He said, "I know you've been working with the handicapped and we're starting a new program at the Center. We're hiring all new staff and I'd like you to consider working there. I know you're well qualified for the position." Needless to say, I was very pleased. This time around I *was* the best qualified of other applicants because of my experience.

I also felt it was the right time for me to make a career move. I had the school program in place and had accomplished everything I set out to do. I was ready for a change and a new challenge.

Meeting the Challenge

It was in this position as senior dental hygienist that I met Dr. Alan Stark who had been appointed chief of dental services. Also on staff were two dental assistants and another dental hygienist.

We were all based in a public institution where the residents historically had had very little dental care. These people were only taken care of in full-blown emergencies; obvious abscesses where extractions were the answer. There was almost no maintenance.

The state had recently undergone a "housecleaning." The head of this facility had been fired, we were hired and we designed a new dental clinic and got it going. It took about a year to build and equip the clinic. While waiting for this to be completed, we surveyed the population, assessed the needs, determined our priorities—and spent much of our time doing oral surgery!

Because of Dr. Stark's background, we were able to do most of the work on site, but when the patients were uncooperative or the work was very extensive, we coordinated our efforts with an urban hospital. That's where I got my training working in the operating room.

157

The Feeling Returns

About three years later, I was starting to feel that it was time for me to move on in my career. At the same time, Dr. Stark was thinking of starting a private practice working with the handicapped.

One of the events tripping off this reaction in each of us was that de-institutionalization was taking place. This meant residents were being moved out of the facility and into the community. We saw that a private specialty practice could fill the needs of this population. Serving that need seemed an ideal way for me to tie together my public health background and my experiences with the handicapped.

Working With the Special Patient

I've been associated with the practice of Dr. Stark for the past four years. We specialize in general dentistry, geriatric dentistry, and dentistry for the handicapped. Although patients are treated in our specially-designed office, we also provide general dental services for the homebound and chronically ill in nursing homes.

About sixty percent of the practice is devoted to general dentistry, 30 percent to the geriatric and handicapped and about ten percent for the homebound. It is these last two areas which utilize my special clinical training and organizational skills. My primary role is that of coordinator of special services interacting with available resources, patients' families, and our treatment plans.

Specifically, since we do extensive work in the hospital, I coordinate the operating room cases re OR time, getting consent from the primary care physician, and sending letters to family members. When we are involved with a homebound patient, I am liaison between the office, the family, third party payors, and confer with Dr. Stark on the treatment plan regarding arrangements and priorities.

I usually accompany and assist Dr. Stark on private residence and nursing home visits and prepare his armamentaria in advance. This depends on the operative procedures to be performed.

For example, if we have to do an endodontic procedure, I would make sure we had the following items in the black bag: sterilized instruments and materials, rubber gloves, face masks, a small flashlight, cotton rolls, bibs, hand towels, and an electronic apex locator. (We often use this in lieu of X-rays in endodontic cases.) If X-rays are a must, we work with a mobile radiographic service. I hand carry the instrument tray and patient's chart.

Our portable equipment for air and water sources is self-contained and designed for out-of-office use. Since both the office and the building are wheelchair-accessible, it is easy for us to roll the carrier out of the office, into the elevator, and down the ramp leading to the parking lot.

Personal Growth

I often feel like a combination RDH and social worker. What starts with a toothache for a handicapped person can often unveil other problems within the family that are not being addressed. It's surprising how often a family locks itself up to the point where they don't know where to turn for help. Through caring about the whole person, I've been able to offer guidance and resources to the family unit so that other health professionals can become involved. It's quite a feeling to be able to help both dentally and in other areas of care as well.

I'm currently taking courses in practice management as I include managing of the office in my goals. I would like a part-time RDH to work with me, Dr. Stark and the dental assistant in the clinical portion of our program while I work with the receptionist to develop the marketing and business aspects of the practice.

Words of Advice

For those hygienists wanting to direct their skills towards working with the mentally and/or physically handicapped patient, I would offer the following advice: Take a continuing education course on dentistry for the handicapped so you'll know what you're getting into. You'll have a better idea of what you'll be encountering.

Also, contact your local chapter of the Association for Retarded Citizens (ARC). Offer to work as a volunteer. Demonstrate your value to the administration. If this is where your interest lies, pursue it. It is very emotionally rewarding but you should understand clearly what you're getting into before you plunge in.

[RDHs interested in contacting Mary Jean can do so directly c/o Dr. Alan Stark, The Wildwood Medical Center, 10401 Old Georgetown Rd., Suite 403, Bethesda, MD 20814. Tel. (301) 530-2700.]

RDH as Office Coordinator

Julie Vaughan outlines her shift from clinical tasks to managerial responsibilities in the private practice environment.

Technology has impacted the dental profession in two distinct aspects during this past decade. One, quality patient care requires thorough diagnosis, organized treatment planning, skilled restoration, proper maintenance, and meticulous record keeping. Two, profitable practice requires production information to establish reasonable goals and fees and to continually monitor practice health.

Understanding marketing, accounting, law, personnel management and clinical treatment are necessary to effectively combine patient care and business management. As computers are installed in more offices each year, a new language is being spoken in dental business offices. And it is spreading to the operatories.

The level of organization, internal and external marketing are all being refined to keep pace with advancing clinical methods and skill. It is the rare dentist who loves to organize, deal with personnel problems, and control the details of running the practice. Dentists are and should be primary care providers. Therefore they need someone else to handle the organization.

The most frequent question asked of me in my present position as office coordinator is, "Where do I look for a good office manager?" My own evolution from a "no previous experience necessary" on-the-job-trained chairside assistant to coordinator of a four-doctor solo group practice, prompts me to suggest first, consider an *enthusiastic* dental hygienist—especially one who has also had chairside experience.

How it Began

In 1976 I began working with Dr. Peter Dawson and Dr. Reuben Roach, two exceptional restorative dentists and organized practice administrators whose practice is located in St. Petersburg, Florida.

Every "go-fer" job was mine; each was expected to be performed perfectly. This taught me the value of all the details which make the difference in producing quality and the patient's perception of the dentist's skill.

It was the era of time in motion and four-handed dentistry. Eventually, chairside duties were added to my job description, and it was there that real quality care was defined. Thorough examinations were then, as now, the basis of all treatment.

160

Patient education and careful maintenance remain the primary objective for providing long-term oral health. Today these two axioms are my principles for office management. First look at the total picture, get all the information, then modify where necessary and monitor the changes.

Getting More Skills

In 1981, I returned to college to get my degree in dental hygiene. My purpose was to *understand* rather than mechanically perform tasks.

Training in patient management and the psychological aspects of patient motivation extend quite naturally into personnel management. It is essential for a successful and happy dental hygienist to be a "people person". An office manager also needs to be a motivator and a trainer, capable of assessing needs and organizing action plans which achieve results. Most important, just as a hygienist probes and measures results, a manager must realize that constant monitoring is an important aspect of reaching long term practice goals.

In preparing to graduate from dental hygiene training, the opportunity to return to Dr. Dawson's and Dr. Roach's practice as a chairside assistant/part-time hygienist was presented to me. The unique position involved initial patient contact and schedule control, assisting with assessment and coordinating preliminary mouth preparation, participating chairside with reconstruction procedures, and designing home care regimen and periodic recall monitoring. This is an optimum level of dental hygiene practice which contributes directly to patient trust and motivation plus a sense of success for the dental team when case completion is accompanied with ongoing patient appreciation.

The Practice Grows

When the need for an office manager with a total vision and understanding of the practice's philosophy arose, the doctors, then totaling four partners, offered the position to me.

There were positive and negative aspects to the promotion. The obvious pluses were increased compensation accompanied by the gratification of vote of confidence in my ability to do the job. The negatives were a surprise.

Friends and co-workers were not sure of the new role and weren't entirely receptive to the change. Also, direct contact with patients decreased, which was a personal loss to me and caused some confusion among loyal patients.

161

The basic job description originally included re-evaluating all departments and recommending organizational changes, clarifying job descriptions and developing evaluation procedures which coordinated with each position, hiring new staff, supervising training and dismissing when necessary, monitoring appointment scheduling and production controls, planning training sessions and postgraduate opportunities, organizing weekly office executive meetings and staff planning time, and being available to substitute for any absent staff member.

Past experience in all areas provided insight and understanding for each position, its contributions, potential and needs.

Time management became the biggest challenge in working with a four doctor, twenty-plus staff. Trial and error became the teacher of valuable lessons in prioritizing and delegation of responsibilities.

More formal training in business management through seminars has been of great benefit in understanding legal and employee relations. Computer training sessions and guidance in utilizing data have increased efficiency in monitoring practice administration and increased internal and external marketing techniques. All these have been accomplished attending evening or weekend classes.

How I Feel Now

My position is more challenging and much more rewarding as organization has increased. Additional patient duties allow interaction with all departments, and thus the opportunity to monitor patient care and needs for improvement. I keep a steady finger on the pulse of the practice.

There is no place for burnout in dental hygiene careers; only a place for increased participation and redirection. The opportunity to advance is unlimited either through on-the-job expansion or by a more structured continuation of postgraduate education.

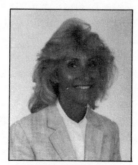

Julie Vaughan

RDH in General Practice

Rosemary Minervini *explains how her years of experience in the profession qualifies her for the challenge of a quality practice.*

I never thought I'd be back in private practice—but I am. And with no regrets whatsoever!

While working in a health maintenance corporation for the past three years, I gained valuable experience in both management and clinical skills for periodontally-involved patients. Although I reached the top of the salary range, I found I needed more stimulation to keep me going.

Not wanting to let"burnout" get to me, I made a list of things I would look for in finding a new position. It included; *control* over working hours, patient scheduling, salary, benefits, operatory equipment, types and numbers of patients, and provide opportunity for growth through professional challenges. With my considerable experience and education, I knew that I could offer an office increased patient flow and productivity.

I started my search by asking other hygienists if they knew of offices needing an experienced RDH. After receiving several good leads and having interviews with several dentists, I accepted a position that offered what I was looking for.

The Industry Calls

At the same time, I was asked to be a consultant by a major dental products manufacturer. This was an opportunity I found most fascinating. My work would be to test and critique new dental products, approach dental schools with grant moneys to formulate and conduct research on new dental products, and represent the company at various dental hygiene and dental conventions to promote their products. Of course I accepted their offer!

Being an industry consultant isn't a full-time position. I do it in addition to my private practice responsibilities. This makes for a very busy schedule which is exactly how I like it.

163

New Products

Since my return to private practice, I designed a new dental chart which is customized to meet our practice's needs.

The front of the chart shows all information on that particular patient for up to ten recall visits. It's concise, accurate and informative. It seems to be a breakaway from the universal charts so traditionally used.

For the elementary schools in the area, I developed a dental health program. I certainly have been pleased with its reception. Not only are the students interested in learning about oral hygiene, but I've been surprised with their inquiries as to how one becomes a dentist or dental hygienist.

Because of an increased interest by the public in general regarding periodontal disease, I developed a dental hygiene periodontal program for my patients. While the program has been in effect only a short while, its success is overwhelming.

As patients become aware of gum disease, they are more than willing to accept treatment. Of course we don't play hero with patients who have severe periodontal disease; they are referred immediately to a periodontist. But for those with beginning to moderate symptoms, the overall change in oral hygiene awareness and health is fantastic!

I've seen 6 mm. pockets reduce to 3 mm. and inflamed tissue return to normal. Patient flow has increased at least 15 percent and dental hygiene production has more than doubled since the program's inception. This is one of those cases where "both sides of the coin" are positive: office production is extremely favorable and the patients are receptive and appreciative of their treatment.

Not "Just a Job"

We all hear of hygienists who go into private practice and within the first few months decide that it's "just a job."

You go to work, clean teeth and then go home. If that's all they do, then I'm sure it *is* "just a job" with nothing to interest or challenge them.

Being involved with dental hygiene since 1970, I have yet to find the profession lacking interest or challenge. The reason is quite simple: I *work* at keeping it interesting and challenging. I can assure you that since I returned to a solo practice, there has never been a dull moment.

How We Function

While it may seem elementary, teamwork is an important ingredient in the operation of an efficient and productive office. In order for teamwork to function properly, everyone has to know what's going on.

Each morning before our patients arrive, we hold a fifteen-minute staff meeting during which the daily schedule is reviewed and goals are set. All cases are discussed which is an added advantage because it eliminates any confusion and adds continuity.

By the time the first patient arrives, we are aware of the treatment plan for each of the 30 patients we average each day.

In addition, we hold a one-hour office meeting every Thursday in which any questions, comments, suggestions or office policies are discussed.

In this practice, we set production goals on a daily, weekly and monthly basis. If we meet or exceed the *weekly* goal, the dentist takes us all out to lunch for our Thursday meeting. If we meet or exceed our *monthly* goal, the entire staff receives a bonus pay check based on a percentage of the profits.

Continuing education is provided to all the staff in order to keep abreast of the latest in the dental profession. As an added incentive, we receive a cash coupon that can be used for continuing education travel expenses for each patient we refer to the office.

Additional benefits include medical and term life insurance, paid vacations and holidays, paid sick days, and profit sharing.

Making it Work Better

Let me talk about another ingredient that goes into the operation of a successful dental office—public relations. At our office we give it top priority because it has paid huge dividends in many ways, not the least of which are referrals.

Here are some examples of the things we do:

— Every week each staff member gives a gift to a patient who was either fun to work with or someone who made a delightful stay of their visit.

— We send greeting cards to patients for special occasions.

— Holidays are celebrated with gifts.

— Flowers are given to each patient as they leave the office.

— People who move into the area are sent "newcomer" letters offering a free prophy and exam. This marketing activity has generated as many as 60 new patients each month, several of whom I've met and treated at other offices.

As with any job, it's what you want to make of it. I've worked in many aspects of dental hygiene, including teaching, research and research writing, consulting, management and clinical practice. All were building blocks to gain additional experience within the profession. All have served as a growth process within my career.

Dental hygienists in private practice uninteresting? No challenge? Boring? "Just a job?"

Hardly!

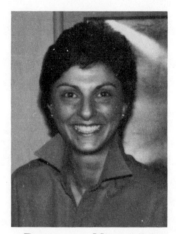

Rosemary Minervini

RDH in General Practice

Anne E. Gwozdek *shares her enthusiasm and professionalism for her career in private practice.*

A common denominator in the career of most dental hygienists is involvement in a clinical capacity within a private dental practice. I have been such a hygienist since 1973 and I love it!

My career began with my graduation from the University of Michigan and since then I have found my position within private practice very satisfying. In addition to fine financial remuneration and benefits, my scheduling freedom has provided the reward of a flexible life style for my husband and myself. Allow me to share with you what I have found to be successful employment in private practice.

Why I Selected Dental Hygiene

One of the principle reasons I originally pursued a career in dental hygiene is that it is such a people-oriented health care profession. I have found that patients can be far more than a clinical challenge. Becoming familiar with patients as people first and always striving to give them the best total oral care is one of the finest ways to a successful patient-RDH relationship.

The open line of communication that you, the hygienist, can develop, permits individualized treatment and education for each patient. I have found that when patients feel you really care about them and their oral health, their response will bring you terrific satisfaction. Realistically, every patient is not a success story, but this, too, can be a challenge in learning to relate to people of different ages and backgrounds.

A Special Environment

The primary reason I have found it possible to develop special rapport with patients comes from my gratifying employment with solo practitioner, James G. Nagy, D.D.S., for the past eleven years. It has been a privilege to be a member of his staff.

Office philosophy is dedicated to a common-sense approach to patient care and prevention concepts. Education for patients and staff is encouraged and ideas and input are always shared. Importance is

167

placed on keeping all staff members updated on patients' case progress. The practice is constantly growing and it is thrilling to be an integral, contributing part of that growth.

Other Opportunities

Through volunteering my dental hygiene services at a public health facility, a part-time position was created for me. I was able to accept this challenge because of my flexibility at Dr. Nagy's office.

This clinic was developed to serve children who had been placed in foster care homes. This was the first dental care facility for this agency, and for many of the children, their first exposure to dentistry.

Many of the children were from an unstable home environment which contributed to a multitude of emotional and behavioral problems. Coordinating their dental care included consultation with medical personnel, and the education process extended to the foster parents and social workers as well as the children. The facility is still in existence today having expanded to include specialty services. (I was involved in the initial establishment of the facility itself including staffing and scheduling.)

Another avenue that has provided me with an opportunity to increase my technical expertise as well as expose me to alternate career directions has been through active participation in association activities.

Involvement, especially at the state and component levels, has introduced me to other RDHs who practice in a variety of settings.

Membership has also given me the chance to take continuing education courses and subscribe to current professional literature. Taking advantage of membership benefits has helped enormously to promote my professional and personal growth.

My active participation has ranged from committee chairperson to president to editor. These positions have helped me to expand my organizational, administrative and creative skills. The rewards that come from involvement have far outweighed the expenditure of time and energy necessary to accomplish the organization's goals.

What Private Practice Can Mean

Private practice dental hygiene entails so much more than "just cleaning teeth." If you accept the challenge to pursue this career direction, always continue to develop your hygiene background.

Find employment in a dental practice where you are a member of a professional team. Your satisfaction will be reflected both professionally and personally.

There are enormous opportunities for growth available in private practice if you are willing to experience and expand your dental hygiene horizons.

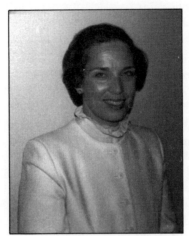

Anne Gwozdek

*[Anne E. Gwozdek can be contacted c/o **Career Directions**.]*

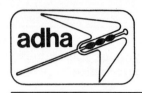

American Dental Hygienists' Association
444 North Michigan Avenue, Suite 3400
Chicago, Illinois 60611 (312)440-8900

Open Letter to Students of Dental Hygiene

Dental hygiene is similar to all other occupations in that there are issues that must be continually addressed. As a practitioner, you need to plan carefully for your future. You need to establish your goals and develop objectives for attainment of those goals.

Dental hygienists currently in practice have been challenged by economic concerns, changes occurring in the delivery of preventive dental services, the need for employment benefits, deviations in work schedules, availability of full-time employment, and regulatory changes.

To protect and enhance your future in the profession, you must become knowledgeable of employee's rights such as workmen's compensation, unemployment benefits, rights as they affect termination, employment contracts (written and verbal), negotiating techniques, and business terminology (overhead, sick leave, personal days, vacation, personnel manual, office policy manual, etc.)

Now is the time to chart your own course. Realize that health care is a "big business" and that the role of the dental hygienist is a separate and distinct profession with the primary function of providing dental oral health.

Because of technological advances that have taken place within the dental delivery system, dental hygienists must be aware of and plan their own destiny. This can be done through personal involvement in your professional association.

Dental hygienists not only have professional responsibilities that must be addressed upon graduation, but a personal obligation to safeguard their lifestyles.

Up until graduation, the majority of students have been nurtured by parents, teachers, guardians or mentors. Now they face the future with all its realities.

Protect your livelihood with proper insurance coverage, both medical and professional liability. Develop a financial reserve plan. Determine where to practice and where to live. Establish a line of credit and open a bank account.

The data reveal dental hygiene is predominantly a woman's profession. But even with all the women's liberation movement's efforts involving working conditions and credit, we find women are being discriminated against when a female RDH becomes a single parent, a widow or is divorced.

Difficult circumstances ensue when credit has not been established in the individual's name. Similarly, a male dental hygienist should maintain a good credit rating.

Research has determined dental hygienists to be dedicated, caring and committed individuals. The role you are assuming in providing preventive oral health care for the public places demands on you both professionally and in your personal life.

Carry out your dedication to the profession by supporting organized dental hygiene through membership in the American Dental Hygienists' Association.

Best wishes to you over the coming years.

> The Membership Staff of the American
> Dental Hygienists' Association

Tear here

Send to: ADHA
444 No. Mich. Ave., Suite 3400
Chicago, IL 60611

Yes. I am interested in becoming a member of the ADHA. Please send an application packet to

Name _____

Street _____

City, State, Zip _____

Résumés That Get
the Interview

How to Write an Effective Résumé

Scenario: You are an employment manager who sees many un-solicited résumés each day. To which of the following two examples would you respond favorably if there were no immediate position open? To which would you respond favorably even if there were an opening?

> JOB OBJECTIVE: I am presently attending a health administra-tion program. I am seeking a position with your organization as a dental administrator.
> JOB OBJECTIVE: To obtain a position that will enable me to use my creative, analytic, and written skills to foster personal and organizational growth.

Probably the first one on both counts, right? Why? Because the writ-er has identified her *purpose* in contacting your organization/company/institution/practice.

Personnel managers, office administrators, department heads, sales managers, people in decision-making positions, are not career counselors. They don't have the time or skill to figure out where anyone's talents could best be utilized in their organization. Their job is to decide *if* the applicant fits, not *where.*

That is why it is so important to identify your *job objective* right up front. It will not be to your advantage to be vague and general in the hope that the person reading your résumé will consider you for more than one position. You will be thought of as having no *purpose* in contacting them.

Getting the Competitive Edge

Put yourself again in the résumé receiver's place. How would you respond to résumés from people you didn't know who were not able to communicate their value to you? You would probably say, "Now what does this person want? Yes, of course, a job. But doing what? I don't have the time to figure it out."

How much better to send a résumé that describes the position you want and presents your achievements as evidence of your competen-cy to do the job.

Everybody has achievements, accomplishments of which they're proud. Make a list of those in which you came out on top. Now think them through carefully and relate them to your goal.

Be timely. You came in first in Girl Scout cookie sales and you're applying for a sales position. Granted that achievement is "related" to your job objective, but unless you're about to graduate from high school, it really isn't appropriate. Your part-time Mary Kay, Amway, Christmas selling, or fund-raising efforts for your church or hygiene component have much more clout.

Do you think you have to write a new résumé for each job you apply for? Not necessarily. Narrow your goals to a field—sales, office management, public relations, hospital administration, whatever—and concentrate your energies within that area. Your *cover letter,* not your résumé, will individualize each situation. (See section on cover letters.)

Let's return to the example in the scenario. Couldn't that job objective in the first example work in a variety of environments: HMOs, retail dental centers, colleges, hospitals, private offices, clinics? Sure it could. The applicant didn't have to write six different résumés.

Targeting Your Recipient

A word of caution regarding unsolicited résumés. Don't count too heavily on "floating" résumés to be read or filed for future consideration "in case something opens up." Most personnel departments are too busy with their immediate workload to give more than cursory attention to that which they "might need some day."

Instead, direct your unsolicited résumé to the person in a decision-making position for the organization in which you would like to work. To make sure your letter reaches the right executives, research *Standard & Poor's Register of Corporations, Directors and Executives* available at your library. It lists 37,000 firms alphabetically along with the addresses and titles of those management personnel you should be contacting.

Bear in mind that many companies are so large that an undirected letter could float around for days, weeks even, before landing on the desk of someone who knows what to do with it. But the primary advantage of doing such a targeted mailing is that you have *narrowed your competition.*

There is often such a super-abundant response to an advertised job that it's hard to get the competitive edge. It may not be your résumé that's at fault; it's just that it is logistically impossible for a company to follow up on everybody.

Résumés That Get Interviews

A résumé has one purpose: to get you an interview which leads to the job. Jobs come through people, not paper.

Your résumé is a statement of what you would like to do as it meets employers' needs, supported by what you have done as it meets employers' needs, in language employers would understand.

Employers are impressed by the *amount* and *kind* of responsibility you have dealt with, not a list of your duties. They want to know the *results* you have achieved and they want to know how those accomplishments you've identified will help them with their present needs.

Contents

Outline your strengths, skills, achievements as it relates to—yes, you guessed it—your *purpose,* your job objective. This gives you the opportunity to list your achievements and how you solved problems, got results. It's called *experience,* regardless of whether it was voluntary or financially-rewarded work. Nobody has to know you didn't get paid for your volunteer work at the local nursing home or for doing oral screenings at the health fair unless you tell them. If you have organizational and administrative skills and are interested in developing them, identify them.

Let's rephrase some of the more common skills and abilities particular to dental hygienists to see if they can be made more pointed.

•Did you "plan treatments and provide complete prophylxis" (responsibility)? Or did you "initiate a patient education program which reduced the DMF rate and rate of gingival inflammation by one-third?" (achievement and problem-solving)

• Did you "purchase supplies and handle accounts receivable?" Or did you "change ordering and inventory control system to achieve a 20 percent cost reduction" and "implemented new billing procedure to reduce outstanding accounts by nearly 30 percent."

• Did you "change the recall system," or "revamped the recall system so that patient visits were increased by 17 percent from the previous year?" Figures, often equated with money, speak louder than words.

Now your prospective employer knows what you can do, what *value* you will be to him for fifty weeks of the year.

The Right Words

Use action words such as initiated, executed, handled, supervised, coordinated, designed: these verbs always take an object and imply a result (initiated *what?* handled *what?* supervised *whom?*)

176

Stay away from the passive voice as in "responsibilities included . . ." For example, "Seventeen new dental hygienists were recruited by me for our local component" is considerably less effective than "I initiated a recruiting program for our local component which resulted in 14 new members, bringing our membership to one of the highest in the state. I am now chairperson of the state membership committee."

Less impressive: "Made crafts for our church/component/school Health Fair."

More impressive: I made crafts which netted the _____ organization $700 in a two-day sale."

Less impressive: Volunteer, handicapped children.

More impressive: Planned and supervised oral health program for 30 handicapped children.

Aren't you proud of your accomplishments? Spell them out! Good work that produces results doesn't need embellishment through overstuffed language to get its message across. And don't be afraid to use the pronoun, "I." Who else did these things?

Now, if you are a new graduate, your work experience is probably limited. You will want to focus on your education and related experiences.

Education

Now is the time to list all your academic accomplishments, honors, and awards. Eliminate class standing unless you were right up there at the top. If your undergraduate work was exceptional, identify which accolades you received.

Other Experience

For an employer, this could be the place where he is sold on you. Many practitioners and administrators feel it is easier to develop clinical expertise than to fill in the personality blanks. What other courses did you take in school? To which organizations and professional associations do you belong? What are your leadership skills, your "people" experiences that round out your character? Assert yourself as a total and whole personality.

Personal Statements

Here is where you state your leisure interests, hobbies, health, marital status, indicate references are available on request, salary negotiable, availability for relocation (if true), and other pertinent information.

Do not include controversial information (divorced, unemployed, let go from last job). Do not say what your husband or parents do. Do not give reference names and addresses unless specifically requested. Do not offer any negative information. (If you think it might be taken the wrong way, it's negative information.) Do not list your Social Security number, height, weight, or age.

Format

People tend to think there is a single way in which to form the information in their résumés. Not so. Your job objective and the statements backing it up are your priority items and should be paramount. If that means highlighting your work experience ahead of your education, so be it. If you are a new graduate with limited experience, lead with your academic accomplishments. It's the *focus* that's important. Whatever your structure, try to keep the sentences short and tight.

Your name and address should hit the eye first (leave the word "résumé" off;' what else could it be?) Use heavy white or off-white paper on an electric typewriter or offset printing. No carbons, cheap duplicating paper, or dot-matrix printing.

Single space with wide margins on sides and bottom (lots of space). Check for grammatical errors and misspellings. Better yet, get someone else to check.

Do not make any strikeovers or whiteouts, and keep your résumé to 1½ pages in length.

Calligraphy, personal stationery or photographs are eye-catching, but they don't *influence.* A well-thought-out presentation on paper is all the influence you need.

How You Can Tell if Your Résumé is Good

If your résumé gets you interviews, it's good. Also, you will be told. People might not tell you they don't like your résumé, but they will tell you if they do. And don't be afraid to use the résumés. They're not supposed to last forever. They're only as good as your next position.

A lot goes into a well-written, effective résumé. A lot of thought. And you must do the thinking. You can go to an outside source for corroboration, but gut-searching is your responsibility.

Who Gets the Job?

Jobs do not go to people with the longest résumés written in the most eloquent language based on inflated experiences. *The best test is that you can talk about anything on your résumé with ease.*

And don't forget that the person reading your résumé is human. She, undoubtedly, has agonized over her own résumé at some point in her career. Perhaps the one that got her the job reading yours! Make it easy for her to say, "This person knows what she wants and what she can deliver."

For Examples of Résumés, Please Turn Page

New Graduate

_____

_____

_____

_____

CAREER OBJECTIVE:

After receiving licensure, my desire is to work as a dental hygienist for a prevention oriented practice.

PROFESSIONAL EDUCATION;

Parkland College, Champaign, Illinois	1981
Certification in Dental Assisting	
Parkland College, Champaign, Illinois	1987
Associate in Applied Science Degree - Dental Hygiene	

CLINICAL EXPERIENCE:

During my clinical courses I became proficient in the following aspects of patient care:
Providing extra-oral and intra-oral examinations, charting, periodontal charting, periodontal probing, oral hygiene home care instruction, exposing and developing radiographs, hand scaling, ultrasonic scaling, root planing, polishing tooth surfaces, and administering topical fluoride treatments.

Among auxiliary procedures I performed were:
applying pit and fissure sealants, taking impressions and producing study models, removing overhangs on amalgam restorations, polishing amalgam restorations, nutritional counseling, and patient education involving phase contrast microscopy.

I also obtained certification in Cardio-Pulmonary Resusitation and am currently certified.

OTHER EXPERIENCE:

Champaign County Nursing Home	1986

I performed extra and intra-oral examinations including cancer screening, oral hygiene instruction, and cleaning of dentures for residents.

Champaign County Nursing Home	1986

I spoke to a group of daycare participants concerning nutritional principles for the elderly.

Community Christian School   1986
I spoke to a first-grade class concerning plaque control
as it relates to basic brushing techniques and monitoring of diet.

Parkland College   1986
I presented a table clinic for area dental personnel concerning the practice of orthodontics.

Chanute Air Force Base, Rantoul, Illinois   1986
I was granted the opportunity to visit this facility and
observe many varied procedures.

Francis Nelson Health Center, Champaign, Illinois   1987
I provided prophylaxis for regularly scheduled patients
in the dental clinic.

Champaign-Urbana Public Health District   1987
I experienced providing prophylaxis for regularly scheduled patients in the dental clinic.

Dr. Steven W. Seibert, D.D.S., Periodontics Practice   1987
Champaign, Illinois
I visited this practice to observe the many procedures
performed for patients needing periodontal treatment.

Parkland College   1987
I completed a programmed computer course designed
to familiarize the dental hygienist with computer applications in dental office management on the IBM-XT
computer.

LICENSURE:
Anticipated Licensure   August, 1987
National Board Certification   1987
Northeast Regional Board Certification   1987
Certified Dental Assistant   August, 1981-December 1982

WORK EXPERIENCE:
Dental Assistant for a Private General Dental Practice
                              August, 1981-August, 1985
Dinah's Hallmark Shop, Champaign, Illinois   1983-85
Cashier and stockperson
Valu-Check Foods, Champaign, Illinois   1985-86
Cash register operator, office personnel
Family Tree, Inc., Champaign, Illinois   1986-present
Sales person, Cashier, compute daily sales reports

PROFESSIONAL ACTIVITIES:

Student American Dental Hygiene Association Active Member	1985-87
National Children's Dental Health Month Active Involvement	1986
Chairman of Parkland College Presentation	1987
District VII Student/Faculty Conference, Chicago, IL Member of table clinic production and luncheon production committees.	1987

Professional and personal references available upon request.

New Graduate

_____
_____
_____
_____

PROFESSIONAL OBJECTIVE:

My professional objective is to utilize my expanded function training within the clinical setting.

PROFESSIONAL EXPERIENCE:

Channel 9 Health Fair Oral Examiner Montbello High School	April 1987
Clinical Research Study Assistant University of Colorado Health Sciences Center	March 1987- May 1987
Clinical Research Study Assistant University of Colorado Health Sciences Center	November 1986- December 1986
Bookshelver University of Colorado Health Sciences Center, Denison Memorial Library	June 1986- April 1987
Dental Assistant Park Central Dental Group Denver, Colorado	November 1984- March 1986
Dental Assistant DentaHealth of Colorado Denver, Colorado	July 1983- November 1984
Peer Advocate University of Colorado at Denver	January 1983- June 1985
Waitress/Hostess Mr. Steak Restaurant Westminster, Colorado	November 1979- August 1985

PROFESSIONAL EDUCATION:

University of Colorado Health Sciences Center
Bachelor of Science Degree

University of Colorado at Denver
Obtained prerequisites for Dental Hygiene School

LICENSURE:

National Written Boards
March 1987

Central Regional Boards
June 1987

State Dental Hygiene License
June 1987

EXPANDED FUNCTION TRAINING:

Administration of local anesthesia, C.P.R., Sealant Application, Alginate impression taking, Curettage, Nutritional Counseling, Placement of amalgam restorations in prepared teeth.

EXTRAMURAL TRAINING:

Includes working the National Foundation of Dentistry for the Handicapped, Health Intervention Program for the Elderly (HIPE), Denver Public Schools, Denver General Hospital and the VA Hospital.

PROFESSIONAL ORGANIZATIONS:

Colorado State Dental Hygienists' Association
American Dental Hygienists' Association

References available on request.

Experienced: Management

_____

_____

_____

_____

_____

OBJECTIVE   To use my dental hygiene education and skills in an administrative/management position; to promote the role of the dental hygienist and increase public awareness toward good dental health outside the dental office.

EDUCATION   B.S. Dental Hygiene, Oregon Health Sciences University, June 1978.
Pre-Dental Hygiene, University of Oregon, 1974-1976.

EXPERIENCE   *Dental Services Coordinator:* Robison Jewish Home, Portland, Or., January 1983 to present. Established the dental program from the beginning. Direct, coordinate the program; provide dental hygiene services.

Dental Hygienist: Dr. _____
D.M.D. Responsible for the dental hygiene services. Beaverton, Or. 1983-present.

Dr. _____ D.M.D. Portland, Or, 1978-1981. Responsible for the dental hygiene services.

Junior Auxiliary Nurse: Salem Memorial Hospital, Salem, Or., 1970-1974.

PUBLIC SPEAKING/ PRESENTATIONS   OHSU Dental Hygiene Junior Class: 1984, 1985.
PCC Dental Hygiene Senior Class: 1984, 1985.
LCC Dental Hygiene Senior Students and Component Members: 1985.
Salem Dental Hygiene Study Club: 1984.
Portland Dental Hygiene Study Club: 1986.
ADHA Educational Workshop, Louisville, Kentucky: Poster presentation, 1985.
Robison Jewish Home Geriatric Nutrition Symposium: 1986.

AFFILIATIONS/
RECOGNITIONS

Oregon Dental Hygienists' Association: 1978-present.

Portland District Dental Hygienists' Association: 1978-present.
> Delegate: 1979-present.
> President: 1982-1983.
> Vice-President: 1981-1982.

Oregon Dental Hygienists' Association: Dental Health Chairman, 1986-present.

Oregon Dental Hygiene Scholarship and Loan Fund, Inc.: Benefit Chairman, 1982. Raised $2600.

Salem Memorial Hospital: Scholarship, 1974-1978 from Junior Auxiliary Nurse's Scholarship Fund.

Experienced: Clinical

JOB OBJECTIVE:	Clinical and Managerial Dental Hygiene in a Growth-Oriented General Practice

EXPERIENCE:

Clinical

I developed a successful periodontal dental hygiene program for patients with early to moderate stages of periodontal disease. This program has more than doubled patient flow and office production.

I provide total comprehensive patient care to periodontally involved patients including treatment planning, local infiltration anesthesia, nitrous oxide sedation, soft tissue curettage, root detoxification, radiographs, record medical and dental histories, fluoride applications, oral hygiene instructions, and initiate effective recall systems.

Consulting

As a consultant for a dental products manufacturer, I evaluate, critique and write reports on new dental products, approach dental schools with grants monies to formulate and conduct research on new dental products, and represent the company at major dental conventions.

Managerial

Dental Hygiene Department Head, Kansas City Dental Care, Kansas City, Missouri, 1983-1985. Responsible for recruitment, orientation and supervision of five dental hygienists; management and organization of record systems for over 11,000 dental hygiene patients; preparation of monthly/annual inventory and budget requisitions; coordinate and assist in operatory design for expanding office space at both main and satellite clinics.

Dental Hygiene Course Supervisor, Marquette University, Milwaukee, Wisconsin, 1981-1982.

187

Course supervision of five faculty members and seventy-six students. Co-ordinated all course activities, prepared annual budget requisitions for needed materials and equipment; designed courses; conducted classroom and laboratory lectures, discussions, examinations; lead and co-ordinated seminars; clinical instruction involving 154 students; monitored and maintained records of progress, attendence and quality of work.

Research

Currently conducting descriptive and scientific dental hygiene research projects; intra-library searches, literature reviews and grantsmanship. Have served on various committees related to evaluation systems, instrument selection, counseling, self-study committee for University reaccreditation.

Research Laboratory Technician, Texas Tech University, Lubbock, Texas, 1974-1978. Conducted the organization and management of cardiovascular research laboratories in the Physiology Department of the Medical School.

EDUCATION:

M.S. in Dental Hygiene Education, May 1981
University of Missouri-Kansas City
School of Dentistry

B.S. in Dental Hygiene Education, May 1980
University of Missouri-Kansas City
School of Dentistry

A.A.S. in Dental Hygiene, June 1973
Erie Community College-North Buffalo, New York

PUBLICATIONS:

Career Directions for Dental Hygienists. Chapter contributions, two editions, Career Directions Press, NJ.

"Career Directions for Dental Hygienists," newsletter, April, 1984, Career Directions Press, NJ

RDH Magazine, May/June, 1984, Stevens Publishing Company, TX

Journal of General Dentistry, 31(6): 466-468, 1983.

Dental Hygiene, 55(5): 36-41, 1981

In-House Publication, University Press, Kansas City, Missouri, 1979.

Thirteen acknowledgement citations for technical assistance published in various international medical journals.

PERSONAL DATA:

Health excellent, middle 30's, single. I am action-oriented, a quick study eager to stretch beyond what I've already accomplished. Salary negotiable. References on request.

Experienced: Sales

Professional Objective: Sales Representative/Dental Products

Experience: *Private Practice* I have been a dental hygienist in private practice for more than ten years. A high standard of care is very important to me. While working, I

- Designed and implemented a method of periodontal assessment for the purpose of documentation and evaluation for the periodontally involved patient. This resulted in clarification of the disease for the patient and legal protection for the dentist.
- Initiated and established prevention and nutritional counselling programs which created better patient rapport.
- Formulated new ordering procedures resulting in a 5% decrease in material costs.
- Anticipated potential dental problems and promoted treatment plans generating additional revenue for the office.

Marketing
- Director of continuing education for the _____ Dental Hygienists' Association.
- Negotiated contracts for speakers and facilities while remaining below budget limitations.
- Wrote, designed and distributed 900 continuing education brochures. Organized and oversaw registration procedures. All this resulted in a 15% increase in course participants.
- Conceptualized, created and sold crafts netting an additional 9% to personal income.

Education: A.S. in Dental Hygiene, (school, address). President's List all semesters. Cumulative average for all academic and clinical courses, 4.0.

Personal: Excellent health, married, two college-age children. Enjoy biking, swimming, calligraphy, reading. I am self-motivated, disciplined, competitive. Exceptional interpersonal skills. References on request.

Résumé Review

DO:

• Include a short, concise career objective.

• Include only information that is relevant, to the point, and which supports your objective.

• Use brief phrases rather than sentences to describe what you have done, and start with strong effective action verbs such as *supervised, developed, controlled, directed, generated, established, organized, coordinated,* and *initiated.*

• Quantitate accomplishments whenever possible. Show the *amount of dollars* you saved or earned for a practice, the *number of people* involved when you reorganized your recalls, or how you streamlined operations for greater efficiency and productivity.

• Include studies, seminars and professional affiliations that relate to your career goals.

• Keep personal information to a minimum, eliminating marital status and number of children.

• List education *after* your work experience unless applying for an educational position or a new graduate.

• List educational achievements from college forward.

DO NOT:

• Mention why you left your last job.

• Include previous employers' names and addresses. Instead, say "References furnished upon request" at the end of your résumé.

• Include salary history, unless specifically requested.

• Identify marital status, number of children, husband's position, Social Security number, age, height, weight.

How to Write
A Cover Letter

Why A Cover Letter?

The cover letter introduces your résumé. *It shapes the prospective employer's initial impression of you* and determines whether or not he will take the time to read your correspondence.

What a cover letter does is tell a potential employer why you'd like to work in that particular place. The more specific the better. If you are making a career change, now is the time to say so.

> . . . "I want to work at XYZ Dental Associates because I have been involved with professional dental care for years and your name/company/HMO is in the forefront of preventive dentistry/quality products/outstanding health services," etc.

Follow your statement by a paragraph of two or three impressive accomplishments (which are also in your résumé) and related to that particular position (or to your identified job objective if you are not answering an ad.)

Your last paragraph should ask for an interview and say that you will call next week to make an appointment. And then call. (And hope they call you first!)

Keep the letter short, directed, and keyed to that organization. Sign it personally.

(1) **Individualize your correspondence.** Each cover letter must be hand-typed on plain white paper, single-spaced, one page only. You can photocopy your résumé but never a cover letter. It's a good idea to include your address and available phone numbers even though you have them on your résumé.

(2) Unless you are responding to a blind ad or box number, **make every effort to get the name and title of the person to whom you are writing.** "Dear Sir or Madam" or "To Whom It May Concern" is offensive to the recipient. It shows lack of thought. If you are contacting a particular company, organization, hospital, practice, whatever, it's an easy thing to call the switchboard or personnel office for the name and correct spelling of the department head/clinic manager/vice-president. Another method is to use business directories. (See section on résumés.)

(3) **Humanize the recipient of your correspondence.** That's what you do when you personalize your salutation. There's a human being at the other end who wants his name spelled right and his position respected.

Remember that the person reading your letter will be asking himself, "What can this person (you) offer my organization/company/practice/program?" The better you can fine-tune your answer, the better are your chances of getting your résumé read.

INTERVIEWS GET JOBS; THE RÉSUMÉ GETS INTERVIEWS; THE COVER LETTER GETS THE RESUME READ!

Interviews that get the job

Nancy J. Salzmann, *a full-time faculty member at Northwestern University Dental School, is currently pursuing a master's degree in management.*

Preparing for the Interview

Now that you have secured an interview, your hard work begins. In order to ensure a successful interview, you must be well prepared. The time and effort you spend in preparation will be worthwhile when you are offered the job that you want!

Whether applying for a position in a private dental practice or in an alternative health care setting, you will want to be familiar with certain basic strategies that can help you manage and win the interviewing game. An effective résumé and cover letter do a great deal to spark an employer's interest in you, to be sure. Your greatest impact, however, is made during the interview itself. Practice and experience, heighten proficient and polished interviewing skills.

Performing a Self-Assessment

Begin the interview process by performing a self-assessment. Analyze yourself to identify skills and personality traits you have to offer a dental office or a health care organization. Critically assess whether you have the interests and abilities specifically required for the job. Consider your skills, strengths, weaknesses, your short- and long-term career goals and objectives, your personal and professional philosophies and your employment expectations.

Such self-knowledge is important in determining your compatibility with the employment situation. Bear in mind that satisfaction and productivity are closely related to the extent to which the job satisfies your needs.

Conducting Research

It's been said that one reason people are unhappy in their work is that they didn't find out enough about the job before accepting it. Learn as much as you can about the specific activities of the job before actively pursuing it. If the job is within a dental office setting, you may want to check with your colleagues or other employees in the office. If the job is within a large organization, you may want to check published sources available in your local public or college library.

Having information about the employer is helpful since most of your interview will focus on your skills and goals and how they relate to those of the office or organization. In reality, though, anonymous organizations don't hire—*people* do. So get information about the interviewer. Will that person be your immediate boss, as may be the case in a dental office setting? Or is he or she a member of the personnel department as in a large organizational setting such as a hospital?

This information will help you understand the individual interviewing you; you will be able to respond more effectively. Get information about the interviewer from other employees or from your own professional contacts.

It is helpful to organize a file that contains all the information you have gathered about your potential employers. Then you can refer to this information when preparing for subsequent interviews.

Handling Employers' Questions

The interview process should be a mutual exchange of information, inquiry and discussion. It is imperative that you predict what the employer wants to know. Several questions will certainly arise during the interview, questions about your education, your work experience, your career goals, your personality. Anticipate these questions so you can formulate well-planned responses prior to the interview.

Questions You May Want to Ask

Since an interview is considered a mutual exchange of information, assume an active role in the process. In fact, one approach to interviewing suggests that the applicant - not the employer - establish the first line of inquiry. The basic premise here is if you can get the employer to tell you exactly what he or she is looking for, you can position yourself as the candidate who best meets those needs.

Ask questions at appropriate times, being careful not to dominate the interview discussion. Some key questions are

- What are the primary responsibilities of this position? May I have a copy of the job description?
  (If your employer has not written a job description, you might suggest that both of you be involved in its preparation. This way both parties will be cognizant of the specific duties and responsibilities of your position.)
- Do you have a formal performance appraisal system? How is this system structured? How often will I be evaluated?

(This is especially important if your raise is based upon your performance evaluation. In a large organization, knowledge of the evaluation system is useful for your advancement within the organization.)

- Will provisions be made for my personal and professional development? Will you support my attendance at conventions, seminars and continuing education courses?
  (This will give you a clue as to whether the dentist is interested in **your** professional development, as well as his or her own.)

- Will malpractice insurance be provided for me?
  This benefit is very important to you, especially with the increasing amount of malpractice litigation in dentistry.
  (If the dentist does not provide coverage for you, be sure to purchase your own policy.)

- Will I be the first person employed in this position or have there been others? How long were they employed?
  If this is a newly-created position, you may have the opportunity to design your own job. If other hygienists have been previously employed in this same position, you may want to ask about their history, especially the length of employment. (The answer may give you some indication of the level of satisfaction of previous employees with the job and/or the office.)

- Who are the people with whom I will be working? May I talk to some of them?
  Your conversations with the dental assistants or other hygienists in the office can give you a sense of the overall "mood" of the office (positive or negative) and whether the employees seem happy or unhappy with their work environment.

There are other questions you may want to ask if you are pursuing a position in a large organizational setting or alternative health care delivery system, such as a hospital or health maintenance organization (HMO). Such questions as

- Where is the organization going? What are the prospects for future growth and expansion of the organization?

- Why is the position open and how long has it been available? What happened to the last person in the position?

- What is the potential for advancement in the organization? To what positions would I likely progress?

- What training and development will be provided for me? Does the organization support additional formal education?

These tactics can be modified to fit the seting. Again, the key is preparation. Take the time to design your questions carefully, so they are specific for the job you want.

During the latter part of the interview is the best time to ask questions about salary, vacation time, insurance coverage, investment plans, profit sharing plans, retirement plans and other benefits. (A word of caution regarding salary and benefits: If you express an *overwhelming* interest in these areas, you run the risk of alienating your interviewer and losing the position!)

Creating a Positive Impression

Besides providing the interviewer with your résumé, there are a few other interviewing tips you may want to try.
- Be punctual.
- Dress appropriately for the position and the office or organization.
- When greeting the interviewer, smile and extend a firm, steady handshake.
- Be alert to your body language throughout the interview.
- Maintain eye contact with the interviewer.
- Following the interview, thank the interviewer for his or her time and ask when you can expect to hear from him or her.
- Write a "thank you" letter following the interview thanking the interviewer for his or her time and expressing your interest in and enthusiasm about the position.
- Take a few minutes to critique your interview performance. Use the critique to identify ways to improve your performance. You will then be better prepared to face your next employment interview.

Suggested Reading

Beatty, R.H. The Five-Minute Interview: A New and Powerful Approach to Interviewing. New York: John Wiley & Sons, Inc., 1986.

Danna, J. Winning the Job Interview Game: Tips for the High-Tech Era. Briarwood: Palomino Press, 1985.

Darby, M.L. and Bushee, E.J., Comprehensive Review of Dental Hygiene. St. Louis: The C.V. Mosby Company, 1986.

Einhorn, L.J., Bradley, P.H. and Baird, J.E. Effective Employment Interviewing: Unlocking Human Potential. Glenview: Scott, Foresman and Company, 1982.

Krannich, C.R. Interview for Success., Virginia Beach: Impact Publications, 1982.

Kimondollo, P.M. "Interview Aid for Applicants," Quintessence of Dental Technology 9(9): 599-601, October, 1985.

201

INTERVIEW TIPS

Most job-hunters make two mistakes when they are being questioned in an interview. First, they fail to *listen to the question.* As a result, they annoy the interviewer either by answering a question that wasn't asked or by giving out a lot of superfluous information.

Second, and perhaps more important, they attempt to answer questions with virtually no preparation. The glibbest person on earth cannot answer questions off the cuff without damaging her chances of success.

What follows are questions that various surveys have indicated are asked most often, *regardless of the job classification.* Study them carefully, develop appropriate responses. Sitting on a hot seat is no time to wing it.

"WHY DO YOU WANT TO WORK HERE?" Because you have done your homework on the company/practice/school/hospital, you already know why. All you must do is organize your reasons into several short, hard-hitting sentences. "You make the best product on the market today;" "Your management is far-sighted; you will soon be the leader in the industry;" "The programs you have are the best in the area."

"WHY SHOULD I HIRE YOU" The interviewer asking this question does not want a lengthy regurgitation of your résumé. She is interested in testing your poise and confidence. Give her a *short, generalized* summary: "I have the qualifications to do the job that has to be done and my track record proves it," or, "I know this is the job for me and that I will be successful."

"WHAT INTERESTS YOU MOST ABOUT THIS POSITION?" Give a truthful, one- or two-word answer like, "The future;" "The challenge;" "The competitiveness;" "The environment." This kind of answer will force the employer to ask you to explain, giving you yet another opportunity to demonstrate your interest.

"WHAT TRAINING/QUALIFICATIONS DO YOU HAVE FOR A JOB LIKE THIS?" Deliver a short, fact-filled summary of the two or three most important qualifications you have. "I have a background in health care;" "I've demonstrated proven financial skills;" "I'm capable of handling several projects simultaneously;" "I have strong supervisory abilities."

FOR CAREER SHIFTERS

"WHY DO YOU WANT TO CHANGE YOUR FIELD OF WORK?" Before your interview spend one hour to organize your reasons into a written statement. *Memorize* this explanation until you can deliver it cold.

You are going to be asked. Your explanation should include:
— How your previous work experience will contribute to your new career;
— What excites you most about this new field;
— How you came to make this career change decision.

You can talk about being in a dead-end position and locked out of advancement opportunities. You can talk about how your job has become routine, void of learning experience. That's acceptable.

What you *cannot* talk about is that your salary is too low, that you hate your employer or co-workers, that you're bored. You'll come over as a job-hopper and hard to get along with.

"WHAT WOULD YOU LIKE TO BE DOING FIVE YEARS FROM NOW?" They ask this because it's on their list. What they really want to hear is how you view yourself, in their organization, down the road. A safe answer is "In a higher level of management." If you're going for an entry-level job, you can be more specific because you know what the progression for that discipline is. (If you don't, find out before the interview.)

You may not be asked these exact questions, but what you *can* count on is that what they want to know about you will fall into four categories:

1. Why are you here? (Why do you want to work in *this* place?)
2. What can you do for them? (What are your skills and abilities?)
3. What kind of person are you? (What are your goals, values?)
4. How much are you going to cost them? (What is your salary range and does it fit in with theirs?)

EVALUATE

After the interview, ask yourself: What points did I make that seemed to interest the interviewer?. . . Did I present my qualifications well?. . . Did I overlook any that are pertinent to *that* position?. . . Did I pass up clues to the best way to "sell" myself?. . . Did I talk too much? Too little?. . . Was I too tense?. . . Too aggressive?. . . Not aggressive enough?. . . How can I improve my next interview?

Resources for Gathering Information

Sources of Funding for Education

* YOUR COLLEGE

   The Financial Aid Office of your school maintains a file of scholarships, grants and awards offered by private and government agencies. Be sure to check with them first.

* AID FROM UNIONS, RELIGIOUS AND FRATERNAL ORGANIZATIONS

   ☐ Many unions provide aid to members and the spouses, sons and daughters of members. For more information, consult your union, or *The AFL-CIO Guide to Union Sponsored Scholarships and Awards*, available free from the Department of Education, AFL-CIO, 815 16th Street, N.W. Washington, D.C. 20006

   ☐ Most organized religions provide some assistance for members through the synod, council, diocese, etc. Call your local church or synagogue for more information.

   ☐ Many local community organizations, such as the Elks Club, Kiwanis, Rotary Club, and other civic, fraternal or religious groups have created scholarships or aid programs. Ask about them.

* GOVERNMENT PUBLICATIONS

   Higher Education Opportunities for Minorities and Women. Lists 275 loans, scholarships, and fellowships for undergraduate, graduate, and postgraduate students. Many of the opportunities are for all students, not just women and minorities. 103 pp. (1986. ED) **104R, $5.50.**

   Order from the Superintendent of Documents, U.S. Government Printing Office, Wash., D.C. 20402

* LIBRARY RESOURCES

   The following books are probably available at your local public or college library. They will give you in-depth information concerning current scholarship, grant, and loan programs, many of them from private sources:

Lovejoy's Scholarship Guide
Simon & Schuster, Inc.
1230 Avenue of the Americas
New York, N.Y. 10020

You Can Win a Scholarship
Barron's Educational Series, Inc.
113 Crossways Park Drive
Woodbury, N.Y. 11797

Scholarships, Fellowships and Laws
Bellman Publishing Co.
P.O. Box 164
Arlington, Mass. 02174

How and Where to Get Scholarships and Loans
Simon & Schuster, Inc.
Educational Div.
1230 Avenue of the Americas
New York, N.Y. 10020

Foundation Grants to Individuals
The Foundation Center
888 Seventh Avenue
New York, N.Y. 10106

*Guide to Grants, Loans and Other Types of Government
   Assistance Available to Students & Educational Institutions*
Public Affairs Press
419 New Jersey Avenue, S.E.
Washington, D.C. 20003

*Complete Grants Sourcebook for Higher Education
   Public Management Institute*
American Council on Education
One Dupont Circle
Washington, D.C. 20036

**There are other sources of financial aid for postsecondary
education:**

• If you are a veteran, Veterans Benefits may be available. Check with
  your local V.A. office.
• If you are employed, your company may help pay your tuition.
• If you are handicapped, check with your local Vocational Rehabilita-
  tion Office.
• If you are enrolled in a health professions school (medical, dental,
  nursing, or allied health professions) contact:

> U.S. Public Health Service
> Bureau of Health Manpower
> Student Assistance Branch
> Center Building, Room G–23
> 3700 East-West Highway
> Hyattsville, Maryland 20782

Health Career Information

- Health Education: Send $10 for an issue of *Allied Health Education Newsletter* to the Dept. of Allied Health, Education and Accreditation, AMA, 535 N. Dearborn St., Chicago, IL 60610. This newsletter does not include dental hygiene but does describe what is going on in various other health care occupations.

  Or send a check for $25.95 (includes postage) made out to The American Medical Association for the 15th edition of their *Allied Health Education Directory*. Mail to Fulfillment Dept., AMA, Box 10946, OP-220-7, Chicago, IL 60610 or call 312/645-5000.

- The Association of University Programs in Health Administration (AUPHA) has a free brochure listing the names of all accredited programs in health services administration, and, for $12.50, a directory which describes each of the undergraduate and graduate programs in detail. For the 1987-89 directory or brochure, write or call AUPHA, 1911 Ft. Myer Drive, Suite 503, Arlington, VA 22209. Tel. 703/524-5500.

- The 1986 government publication, *Medical and Dental Practitioners and Assistants* gives the employment outlook for chiropractors, dental assistants, RDHs, dentists, medical assistants, etc. For ordering and current pricing, contact the Superintendent of Documents, U.S. Government Printing Office, Washington, D.C. 20402.

- For information on graduate training in research supported by the National Institute of Dental Research, address your request to Special Assistant for Coordination & Training, NIDR, Extramural Programs, Westwood Bldg., Rm. 507, Bethesda, MD 20205.

- The Health Services Administration is that branch of the Public Health Service offering direct health care service to the American public. For further information write to Office of Communications and Public Affairs, Health Services Administration, 5600 Fishers Lane, Rockville, MD 20857.

Federal Job Information Centers (FJICs)

The Office of Personnel Management (OPM) operates FJICs in the cities listed next. FJICs can provide general information on Federal employment, explain how to apply for specific jobs, supply application materials and conduct written examinations, when required.

You can get information by mail, telephone, or by visiting one. The easiest method, if you want information or application materials for a specific job or occupation and can identify it clearly, is to write.

208

The following is a list of the OPM offices which provide Federal job information and testing services.

ALABAMA
Huntsville:
Southerland Building
806 Governors Dr., S.W. 35801
(205) 453-5070

ALASKA
Anchorage:
Federal Bldg. & U.S. Courthouse
701 C St., P.O. Box 22, 99513
(907) 271-5821

ARIZONA
Phoenix:
U.S. Postal Service Bldg.
522 N. Central Ave. 85004
(602) 261-4736

ARKANSAS
Little Rock:
Federal Bldg., Third Floor
700 W. Capitol Ave. 72201
(501) 378-5842

CALIFORNIA
Los Angeles:
Linder Bldg.
845 S. Figueros 90017
(213) 688-3360

Sacramento
1029 J St., Rm. 202 95814
(916) 440-3441

San Diego:
880 Front St. 92188
(714) 293-6165

San Francisco:
211 Main St.,
Second Floor 94105
(415) 974-9725

COLORADO
Denver:
1845 Sherman St. 80203
(303) 837-3509

CONNECTICUT
Hartford:
Federal Bldg., Rm. 613
450 Main St. 06103
(203) 722-3096

DISTRICT OF COLUMBIA
Metro Area:
1900 E Street, N.W., 20415
(202) 737-9616

FLORIDA
Orlando:
Federal Bldg. & U.S. Courthouse
80 N. Hughey Ave. 32801
(305) 420-6148 or 6149

GEORGIA
Atlanta:
Richard B. Russell Federal Bldg.,
9th Floor
75 Spring St. SW, 30303
(404) 221-4315

GUAM
Agana:
Pacific News Bldg.
238 O'Hara St.
Room 308 96910
344-5242

HAWAII
Honolulu (and Island of Oahu):
Federal Bldg., Room 1310
300 Ala Moana Blvd. 96850
(808) 546-8600

ILLINOIS
Chicago:
55 E. Jackson, Rm. 1401, 60604
(312) 353-5136

INDIANA
Indianapolis:
46 East Ohio Street, Room 124, 46204
(317) 269-7161

IOWA
Des Moines:
210 Walnut St., Rm. 191, 50309
(515) 284-4545
In Scott and Pottawattamie Counties
dial (402) 221-3815.

KANSAS
Wichita:
 One-Twenty Bldg., Rm. 101
 120 S. Market St. 67202
 (316) 269-6106
In Johnson, Leavenworth and Wyandotte
Counties dial (816) 374-5702.

LOUISIANA
New Orleans:
 F. Edward Hebert Bldg.
 610 South St., Rm. 103, 70130
 (504) 589-2764

MARYLAND
Baltimore:
 Garmatz Federal Building
 101 W. Lombard St. 21201
 (301) 962-3822
DC Metro Area:
 1900 E St., N.W., 20415
 (202) 737-9616

MASSACHUSETTS
Boston:
 3 Center Plaza, 02108
 (617) 223-2571

MICHIGAN
Detroit:
 477 Michigan Ave., Rm. 595, 48226
 (313) 226-6950

MINNESOTA
Twin Cities:
 Federal Bldg.
 Ft. Snelling, Twin Cities 55111
 (612) 725-4430

MISSISSIPPI
Jackson:
 100 W. Capitol St. (Suite 335) 39260
 (601) 960-4585

MISSOURI
Kansas City:
 Federal Bldg., Rm. 134
 601 E. 12th St. 64106
 (816) 374-5702
St. Louis:
 Old Post Office, Rm. 400
 815 Olive St. 63101
 (314) 425-4285

NEBRASKA
Omaha:
 U.S. Courthouse and Post Office Bldg.
 Rm. 1010, 215 N. 17th St. 68102
 (402) 221-3815

NEW HAMPSHIRE
Portsmouth:
 Federal Bldg., Rm. 104
 80 Daniel St. 03801
 (603) 436-7720 ext. 762

NEW JERSEY
Newark:
 Peter W. Rodino Jr., Federal Bldg.
 970 Broad St. 07102
 (201) 645-3673
In Camden, dial (215) 597-7440.

NEW MEXICO
Albuquerque:
 Federal Bldg., 421 Gold Ave., SW, 87102
 (505) 766-5583

NEW YORK
New York City:
 Jacob K. Javits Federal Bldg.
 26 Federal Plaza 10278
 (212) 264-0422
Syracuse:
 James N. Hanley Federal Bldg.
 100 S. Clinton St. 13260
 (315) 423-5660

NORTH CAROLINA
Raleigh:
 Federal Bldg., 310 New Bern Ave.
 P.O. Box 25069, 27611
 (919) 755-4361

OHIO
Dayton:
 Federal Building
 200 W. 2nd St. 45402
 (513) 225-2720

OKLAHOMA
Oklahoma City:
 200 NW Fifth St., Rm. 205, 73102
 (405) 231-4948

OREGON
Portland:
 Federal Bldg.
 1220 SW Third St. 97204
 (503) 221-3141

PENNSYLVANIA
Harrisburg:
Federal Bldg., Rm. 168, 17108
(717) 782-4494

Philadelphia:
Wm. J Green, Jr. Fed. Bldg.
600 Arch Street 19106
(215) 597-7440

Pittsburgh:
Fed. Bldg., 1000 Liberty Ave. 15222
(412) 644-2755

PUERTO RICO
San Juan:
Federico Degetau Federal Bldg.
Carlos E. Chardon St.
Hato Rey, P.R. 00918
(809) 753-4209

RHODE ISLAND
Providence:
Federal Bldg., Rm. 310
Kennedy Plaza 02903
(401) 528-5251

SOUTH CAROLINA
Charleston:
Federal Bldg., 334 Meeting St. 29403
(803) 724-4328

TENNESSEE
Memphis:
Federal Bldg., 100 N. Main St. 38103
(901) 521-3956

TEXAS
Dallas:
Rm. 6B4, 1100 Commerce St. 75242
(214) 767-8035

Houston:
701 San Jacinto St., 4th Floor, 77002
(713) 226-2375

San Antonio:
643 E. Durango Blvd. 78206
(512) 229-6611

VIRGINIA
Norfolk:
Federal Bldg., Rm. 220
200 Granby Mall 23510
(804) 441-3355

D.C. Metro Area:
1900 E Street, N.W. 20415
(202) 737-9616

WASHINGTON
Seattle:
Federal Bldg., 915 Second Ave. 98174
(206) 442-4365

WEST VIRGINIA
Charleston:
Federal Bldg., 500 Quarrier St. 25301
(304) 343-6181, ext. 226

Uniformed Services Dental Facilities

There can be employment opportunities for dental hygienists in a military setting. Jobs for civilians vary, however, since the Uniformed Services train their own people in preventive skills.

The best way to find out is by calling the Personnel Office of the individual facility to ask if there are openings for civilian dental hygienists in the dental clinic.

ALABAMA
US Army Dental Clinic, Redstone Arsenal, Huntsville 35809

US Army Dental Clinic, Fort Rucker, Enterprise 36362

US Army Dental Clinic, Fort McClellan, Anniston 36205

USAF Dental Clinic, Gunter Air Force Station, 36114-5300

USAF Dental Clinic, Maxwell Air Force Base, 36114-5300

ALASKA
US Army Dental Clinic, Fort Richardson, Anchorage 99505

US Army Dental Clinic, Fort Greely, Big Delta

US Army Dental Clinic, Fort Wainwright, Fairbanks 99703

Dental Clinic, 17th Coast Guard District, Juneau 99802

US Coast Guard Air Station Dental Clinic, Sitka 99835

USAF Dental Clinic, Eielson Air Force Base, 99702-5300

USAF Dental Clinic, Elmendorf Air Force Base, 99506-5300

Fort Wainwright, Fairbanks 99703

Naval Regional Dental Clinic, Adak FPO Seattle 98791

ARIZONA
US Army Dental Clinic, Fort Huachuca, Sierra Vista 85613

US Army Dental Clinic, Yuma Proving Ground, Yuma 85365

USAF Dental Clinic, Davis-Monthan Air Force Base, 85707-5300

USAF Dental Clinic, Luke Air Force Base, 85309-5300

USAF Dental Clinic, Williams Air Force Base, 85224-5300

Naval Branch Dental Clinic, Marine Corps Air Station, Yuma 85369

ARKANSAS
*US Army Dental Clinic, Fort Chaffee, Fort Smith

USAF Dental Clinic, Blytheville Air Force Base, 72315-5300

USAF Dental Clinic. Little Rock Air Force Base, 72099-5300

*Dental clinic closed several months annually.

CALIFORNIA
US Army Dental Clinic, Sierra Army Depot, Herlong 96113

US Army Dental Clinic, Fort Hunter Liggett, Jolon 93928

US Army Dental Clinic, Presidio of Monterey, Monterey 93940

US Army Dental Clinic, Fort Irwin, Barstow 92310

USAF Dental Clinic, Air Force Unit Post Office, Los Angeles 90009-5300

US Coast Guard Dental Clinic, Base Terminal Island, Long Beach 90822

USAF Dental Clinic, Norton Air Force Base, 92409-5300

USAF Dental Clinic, McClellan Air Force Base, 95652-5300

USAF Dental Clinic, Beale Air Force Base, 95903-5300

USAF Dental Clinic, Castle Air Force Base, 95342-5300

USAF Dental Clinic, Edwards Air Force Base, 93523-5300

USAF Dental Clinic, George Air Force Base, 92392-5300

USAF Dental Clinic, March Air Force Base, 92518-5300

USAF Dental Clinic, Travis Air Force Base, 94535-5300

USAF Dental Clinic, Vandenberg Air Force Base, 93437-5300

USAF Dental Clinic, Mather Air Force Base, 95655-5300

Naval Dental Clincs:
  San Diego, CA 92136
  Camp Pendleton, CA 92055
  Long Beach, CA 90822
  San Francisco, CA 94130
Naval Branch Dental Clinics:
  CBC, Port Hueneme, CA 93043
  FLEASWTRACENPAC, San Diego,
  CA 92147
  MCAGC, Twentynine Palms, CA 92278
  El Toro, Santa Ana, CA 92709
  MCAS, (H) Tustin, CA 92710
  MCMWTC, Bridgeport, CA 93517
  MCRD, San Diego, CA 92140
  NAS, Alameda, CA 94501
  NAS, Lemoore, CA 93245
  NAS, Miramar, San Diego, CA 92145
  NAS, Moffett Field, CA 94035
  NAS, North Island, San Diego,
  CA 92135
  NAS, Point Mugu, CA 93042
  NAVCOMSTA, Stockton, CA 95203
  NAVPGSCOL, Monterey, CA 93943
  NAVPHIBASE, Coronado, CA 92155
  NAVSTA, Mare Island, CA 94592
  NAVWPNCEN, China Lake, CA 93555
  NSC, San Diego, CA 92132
  NTC, San Diego, CA 92133
  SUBASE, San Diego, CA 92106
  WPNSTA, Concord, CA 94520
  WPNSTA, Seal Beach, CA 90740
  MCLB, Barstow, CA 92311
  NAF, El Centro, CA 92243
  NCBC, Port Hueneme, CA 93043

COLORADO
US Army Dental Clinic, Fitzsimons, Aurora
80045-5000
US Army Dental Clinic, Fort Carson,
  Colorado Springs 80913-5000
USAF Dental Clinic, Lowry Air Force
  Base, 80230-5300
USAF Dental Clinic, Peterson Air Force
  Base, 80914-5300
USAF Dental Clinic, US Air Force
  Academy, 80840-5300

CONNECTICUT
Branch Naval Dental Clinic, SUBASE New
  London, Groton, CT 06340

DELAWARE
USAF Dental Clinic, Dover Air Force
  Base, 19902-5300

DISTRICT OF COLUMBIA
US Army Dental Clinics:
  Walter Reed, Washington DC
  20307-5000
  Fort McNair, Washington, DC 20319
  Pentagon, Washington, DC 20310
USAF Dental Clinic Bolling, Bolling AFB,
  DC 20332-5300
Naval Branch Dental Clinics:
  NAF, Washington, DC 20390
  NAVSECSTA, Washington, CD 20390
  Navy Yard, Washington, DC 20374
  Arlington Annex, Washington, DC 20370
  Marine Barracks, 8th & I, Washington,
  DC 20390

FLORIDA
US Coast Guard Air Station Dental Clinic
  Clearwater 33520
US Coast Guard Base Dental Clinic, 100
  MacArthur Causeway, Miami Beach
  33139
USAF Dental Clinic, Eglin Air Force Base,
  32542-5300
USAF Dental Clinic, Homestead Air Force
  Base, 33039-5300
USAF Dental Clinic, MacDill Air Force
  Base, 33608-5300
USAF Dental Clinic, Patrick Air Force
  Base, 32925-5300
USAF Dental Clinic, Tyndall Air Force
  Base, 32403-5300
Naval Dental Clinics:
  Jacksonville, FL 32212
  Orlando, FL 32813
  Pensacola, FL 32508
Naval Branch Dental Clinics:
  NAS, Cecil Field, FL 32215
  NAS, Key West, FL 33040
  NAS, Whiting Field, Milton, FL 32570
  NAVCOASTSYSCEN, Panama City, FL
  32407
  NAVSTA, Mayport, FL 32228
  NAVTECHTRACEN, Pensacola, FL 32511

GEORGIA
US Army Dental Clinic, Fort Gordon,
  Augusta 30905-5060
US Army Dental Clinic, Fort Benning,
  Columbus 31905
US Army Dental Clinic, Fort Stewart,
  Savannah 31314-5300

US Army Dental Clinic, Hunter Army
Airfield, Savannah 31409
US Army Dental Clinic, Fort McPherson,
Atlanta 30330
USAF Dental Clinic, Moody Air Force
Base, 31699-5300
USAF Dental Clinic, Robins Air Force
Base, 31098-5300
Naval Branch Dental Clinic, Naval Air
Station, Marietta 30060
Naval Branch Dental Clinic, Marine Corps
Logistics Base, Albany 31704
Naval Branch Dental Clinic, NAVSCSCOL,
Athens 30601

HAWAII
US Army Dental Clinics:
Tripler, Honolulu, Oahu
(Mailing address:
Tripler Army Medical Center, HI
96853-5300)
Schofield Barracks, Honolulu, Oahu
(Mailing address:
Tripler Army Medical Center, HI
96853-5300)
Fort Shafter, Honolulu, Oahu
(Mailing address:
Tripler Army Medical Center, HI
96853-5300)
Pohakuloa Training Center, Hilo, Hawaii
(Mailing address:
Tripler Army Medical Center, HI
96853-5300)
USAF Dental Clinic Hickam, Hickam AFB,
HI 96853-5300
US Coast Guard Base Dental Clinic,
Honolulu, Oahu, HI 96819
Naval Dental Clinic, Pearl Harbor, Oahu,
HI 96860
Naval Branch Dental Clinics:
MCAS, Kaneohe Bay, HI 96863
NAS, Barbers Point, HI 96862
NAVCAMS, East Pac, Wahiawa, HI
96786
NAVMAG, Lualualei, HI 96792
MCB Camp H.M. Smith, HI 96861
PACMISRNG Kekaha Kauai, HI 96752

IDAHO
USAF Dental Clinic, Mountain Home Air
Force Base, 83648-5300
Naval Branch Dental Clinic, Idaho Falls
83402

ILLINOIS
US Army Dental Clinic, Fort Sheridan,
Highwood 60037
USAF Dental Clinic, Scott Air Force Base,
62225-5300
USAF Dental Clinic, Chanute Air Force
Base, 61868-5300
Naval Dental Center, Great Lakes 60088
Naval Branch Dental Clinic, Naval Air
Station, Glenview 60026

INDIANA
USAF Dental Clinic, Grissom Air Force
Base, 46971-5300
US Army Dental Clinic, Fort Benjamin
Harrison, Indianapolis 46216-7000

KANSAS
USAF Dental Clinic, McConnell Air Force
Base, 67221-5300
US Army Dental Clinic, Fort Leavenworth,
66027-5400
US Army Dental Clinic, Fort Riley,
66442-5036

KENTUCKY
US Army Dental Clinic, Fort Campbell,
Hopkinsville 42223
US Army Dental Clinic, Fort Knox,
Elizabethtown 40121

LOUISIANA
US Army Dental Clinic, Fort Polk,
Leesville 71459
USAF Dental Clinic, Barksdale Air Force
Base, 71110-5300
USAF Dental Clinic, England Air Force
Base, 71301-5300
Naval Branch Dental Clinic, New Orleans
70146

MAINE
USAF Dental Clinic, Loring Air Force
Base, 04750-5300
Naval Branch Dental Clinic, Naval Air
Station, Brunswick 04011
Naval Branch Dental Clinic, Naval
Security Group Activity, Winter Harbor
04693
Naval Branch Dental Clinic, Cutler Naval
Communication Unit, East Machias
04630

MARYLAND

US Army Dental Clinic, Fort George G. Meade, Odenton 20755

US Army Dental Clinic, Fort Ritchie, Cascade 21719

US Army Dental Clinic, Edgewood Area, Aberdeen Proving Ground 21005

US Army Dental Clinic, Fort Detrick, Frederick 21701

National Naval Dental Center, Bethesda 20814

Naval Branch Dental Clinic, US Naval Academy, Annapolis 21402

Naval Branch Dental Clinic, Naval Ordnance Station, Indian Head 20640

Naval Branch Dental Clinic, Naval Air Station, Patuxent River 20670

US Air Force Dental Clinic, Andrews Air Force Base, 20331-5300

MASSACHUSETTS

US Army Dental Clinic, Fort Devens, Ayer 01433

USAF Dental Clinic, Hanscom Field AFB, 01730-5300

Naval Branch Dental Clinic, Naval Air Station, South Weymouth 02190

MICHIGAN

Naval Branch Dental Clinic Naval Air Facility, Detroit 48043

USAF Dental Clinic, K.I. Sawyer Air Force Base, 49843-5300

USAF Dental Clinic, Wurtsmith Air Force Base, 48753-5300

MINNESOTA

No dental facilities in this state

MISSISSIPPI

Naval Branch Dental Clinic, Construction Battalion Center, Gulfport 39501

Naval Branch Dental Clinic, Naval Air Station, Meridian 39309

Naval Branch Dental Clinic, Naval Home, Gulfport 39501

Naval Branch Dental Clinic, Supervisor of Shipbuilding, Conversion and Repair, Pascagoula 39567

USAF Dental Clinic, Columbus Air Force Base, Columbus 39701-5300

USAF Dental Clinic, Keesler Air Force Base, 39534-5300

MISSOURI

US Army Dental Clinic, Fort Leonard Wood, Waynesville 65473

US Army Dental Clinic, Federal Building, 1520 Market St., St. Louis 63103

USAF Dental Clinic, Whiteman Air Force Base, 65301-5300

Naval Branch Dental Clinic, Marine Corps Finance Center, Kansas City 64197

MONTANA

USAF Dental Clinic, Malmstrom Air Force Base, Great Falls 59402-5300

NEBRASKA

USAF Dental Clinic, Offutt Air Force Base, 60113-5300

NEVADA

US Army Dental Clinic, Hawthorne Army Ammunition Depot, Hawthorne (Mailing address: Letterman Army Medical Center Presidio of SF, CA 94129-6700)

USAF Dental Clinic Nellis, Nellis AFB, NV 89191-5300

Naval Branch Dental Clinic, NAS Fallon, NV 89406

NEW HAMPSHIRE

Naval Branch Dental Clinic, Naval Shipyard, Portsmouth 03801

USAF Dental Clinic, Pease Air Force Base, 03801-5300

NEW JERSEY

US Army Dental Clinic, Fort Dix, Pemberton 08640

US Army Dental Clinic, Fort Monmouth, Eatontown 07703

USAF Dental Clinic, McGuire Air Force Base, 08641-5300

Naval Branch Dental Clinic, Naval Air Engineering Center, Lakehurst 08733

US Coast Guard Training Center Clinic, Cape May 08204

NEW MEXICO

US Army Dental Clinic, White Sands Missile Range, Las Cruces (Mailing address: William Beaumont Army Medical Center El Paso, TX 79920-5001)

USAF Dental Clinic, Cannon Air Force
Base, 88101-5300
USAF Dental Clinic, Holloman Air Force
Base, 88330-5300
USAF Dental Clinic, Kirtland Air Force
Base, 87117-5300

NEW YORK
US Army Dental Clinic, U S Military
Academy, West Point 10996
US Army Dental Clinic, Fort Hamilton,
Brooklyn 11252
US Army Dental Clinic, Seneca Army
Depot, Romulus 14541
US Army Dental Clinic, Fort Drum,
Watertown 13601
Naval Branch Dental Clinic, Naval
Support Activity, Brooklyn 11251
US Coast Guard Support Center Clinic,
Governors Island, New York City 10004
Naval Branch Dental Clinic,
NAVADMINUNIT, Ballston Spa, NY
12020
USAF Dental Clinics:
Griffiss AFB, NY 13441-5300
Plattsburg AFB, NY 12903-5300

NORTH CAROLINA
US Army Dental Clinic, Fort Bragg,
Fayetteville 28307-5000
USAF Dental Clinic, Pope Air Force Base,
28308-5300
USAF Dental Clinic, Seymour Johnson Air
Force Base, 27531-5300
US Coast Guard Group Dental Clinic,
Fort Macon, Atlantic Beach 28512
Naval Dental Center, Camp Lejeune
28542
Naval Branch Dental Clinic, Marine
Corps Air Station, Cherry Point 28533
Naval Branch Dental Clinic, Marine
Corps Air Station, Jacksonville 28545
US Coast Guard Marine Safety Office
Dental Clinic, Wilmington 28401-3907

NORTH DAKOTA
USAF Dental Clinic, Grand Forks Air
Force Base, 58205-5300
USAF Dental Clinic, Minot Air Force Base,
58705-5300

OHIO
USAF Dental Clinic, Wright-Patterson Air
Force Base, 45433-5300

OKLAHOMA
US Army Dental Clinic, Fort Sill, Lawton
73503
USAF Dental Clinic, Vance Air Force
Base, 73701-5300
USAF Dental Clinic, Altus Air Force Base,
73521-5300
USAF Dental Clinic, Tinker Air Force
Base, 73145-5300

OREGON
US Coast Guard Air Station Dental Clinic,
2000 Connecticut Avenue, North Bend
97459

PENNSYLVANIA
US Army Dental Clinic, Carlisle Barracks,
Carlisle 17013
Naval Dental Center, Philadelphia 19112
Naval Branch Dental Clinic, Naval Air
Station, Willow Grove 19090

RHODE ISLAND
Naval Regional Dental Center, Newport
02841
NAVSUBBASE, New London, Groton
06340

SOUTH CAROLINA
US Army Dental Clinic, Fort Jackson,
Columbia 29207
USAF Dental Clinic, Charleston Air Force
Base, Charleston 29404-5300
Naval Dental Center, Charleston 29408
Naval Branch Dental Clinic, Naval
Weapons Station, Charleston 29408
Naval Dental Center, Parris Island 29905
USAF Dental Clinic, Myrtle Beach Air
Force Base, 29577-5300
USAF Dental Clinic, Shaw Air Force Base,
29152-5300

SOUTH DAKOTA
USAF Dental Clinic, Ellsworth Air Force
Base, 57706-5300

TENNESSEE
Naval Branch Dental Clinic, Millington
38054

TEXAS
USAF Dental Clinic, Brooks Air Force
Base, 78235-5300

USAF Dental Clinic, Goodfellow Air Force Base, 76908-5300
USAF Dental Clinic, Kelly Air Force Base, 78241-5300
USAF Dental Clinic, Randolph Air Force Base, 78150-5300
USAF Dental Clinic, Bergstrom Air Force Base, 78743-5300
USAF Dental Clinic, Carswell Air Force Base, 76127-5300
USAF Dental Clinic, Dyess Air Force Base, 79607-5300
USAF Dental Clinic, Lackland Air Force Base, 78236-5300
USAF Dental Clinic, Laughlin Air Force Base, 78843-5300
USAF Dental Clinic, Reese Air Force Base, 79489-5300
USAF Dental Clinic, Sheppard Air Force Base, 76311-5300
Naval Branch Dental Clinic, Naval Air Station, Corpus Christi 78419
Naval Branch Dental Clinic, Naval Air Station, Dallas 75211
Naval Branch Dental Clinic, Chase Field Naval Air Station, Beeville 78103
Naval Branch Dental Clinic, Naval Air Station, Kingville 78363
US Army Dental Clinic, Fort Bliss, El Paso 79916
US Army Dental Clinic, Fort Hood, Killeen 76544
US Army Dental Clinic, Fort Sam Houston, San Antonio 78234

UTAH
US Army Dental Clinic, Dugway Proving Ground, Dugway
(Mailing address:
Fitzsimons Army Medical Center
Aurora, CO 80045-5000)
USAF Dental Clinic Hill, Hill AFB, UT 84056-5300

VERMONT
No dental facilities in this state

VIRGINIA
US Army Dental Clinics:
Defense General Supply Center, Richmond, VA 23219

Fort A.P. Hill, Bowling Green
(Mailing address:
Dewitt Army Hospital, Fort Belvoir VA, 22060-5166)
Vint Hill Farms Station, Warrenton
(Mailing address:
Dewitt Army Hospital, Fort Belvoir VA, 22060-5166)
Fort Belvoir, Springfield, VA 22060-5166
Fort Monroe, Hampton
(Mailing address:
McDonald Army Hospital
Fort Eustis, VA 23604-5567)
Fort Story
(Mailing address:
McDonald Army Hospital
Fort Eustis, VA 23604-5567)
Fort Eustis, Lee Hall
(Mailing address:
McDonald Army Hospital
Fort Eustis, VA 23604-5567)
Fort Lee, Petersburg, VA 23801-5260
Fort Myer, Arlington, VA 22211
Fort Pickett, Blackstone, VA 23824
USAF Dental Clinic, Langley Air Force Base, 23665-5300
Naval Dental Center, Norfolk 23511
Naval Branch Dental Clinic, Naval Weapons Station, Yorktown 23691
Naval Branch Dental Clinic, Little Creek Naval Amphibious Base, Norfolk 23521
Naval Branch Dental Clinic, Naval Shipyard, Portsmouth 23700
Naval Branch Dental Clinic, Dam Neck Fleet Combat Training Center, Virginia Beach 23461
Naval Branch Dental Clinic, CINCLANFLT Norfolk, 23511
Naval Branch Dental Clinic, Naval Air Station, Virginia Beach 23460
Naval Branch Dental Clinic, Armed Forces Staff College, Norfolk 23511
Naval Branch Dental Clinic, Supervisor of Shipbuilding, Conversion and Repair, Newport News 23607
Naval Branch Dental Clinic, MCDEC, Quantico 22134
Naval Branch Dental Clinic, Naval Surface Weapons Denter, Dahlgren 22443

WASHINGTON
US Army Dental Clinic, Fort Lewis, Tacoma 98433

217

USAF Dental Clinic, McChord Air Force
Base, 98438-5300
Naval Dental Center, Bremerton 98314
Naval Branch Cental Clinic, Whidbey
Island Naval Air Station, Oak Harbor
98278
Naval Branch Dental Clinic, Naval
Support Activity, Seattle 98115
USAF Dental Clinic, Fairchild Air Force
Base, 99011-5300
Makah Air Force Station, Neah Bay
98357
SUBASE Bangor, Bremerton, WA 98315
NAVFAC, Pacific Beach, WA 98115

WEST VIRGINIA
No dental facilities in this state

WISCONSIN
US Army Dental Clinic, Fort McCoy,
Sparta 54656

NOTE: Dental Clinic is closed several
months annually

WYOMING
USAF Dental Clinic, Francis E. Warren Air
Force Base, 82005-5300

Veterans Administration Hospital Locations

VA hospitals at the following locations range in capacity from approximately 100 to over 1,500 beds. Average bed capacity is about 600. Most have general medical and surgical, pulmonary disease, and psychiatric units. Others are predominantly psychiatric. Many have research programs, dental clinics, outpatient clinics or domiciliaries. Contact the Personnel Officer at the individual hospital for specific information on jobs.

ALABAMA
Birmingham 35233
Montgomery 36109
Tuscaloosa 35401
Tuskegee 36083

ALASKA
Anchorage 99501

ARIZONA
Phoenix 85021
Prescott 86313
Tucson 85723

ARKANSAS
Fayetteville 72701
Little Rock 72206

CALIFORNIA
Fresno 93703
Livermore 94550
Loma Linda 92357
Long Beach 90822
Los Angeles (West Los Angeles) 90073
Martinez 94553

Palo Alto 94304
San Diego 92161
San Francisco 94121
Sepulveda 91343

COLORADO
Denver 80220
Fort Lyon 81038
Grand Junction 81501

CONNECTICUT
Newington 06111
West Haven 06516

DELAWARE
Wilmington 19805

DISTRICT OF COLUMBIA
Washington 20422

FLORIDA
Bay Pines 33504
Gainesville 32602
Lake City 32055
Miami 33125
Tampa 33612

GEORGIA
Augusta 30904
Decatur (Atlanta) 30033
Dublin 31021

HAWAII
Honolulu 96813

IDAHO
Boise 83702

ILLINOIS
Chicago (Lakeside) 60611
Chicago (West Side) 60680
Danville 61832
Hines 60141
Marion 62959
North Chicago 60064

INDIANA
Fort Wayne 46805
Indianapolis 46202
Marion 46952

IOWA
Des Moines 50310
Iowa City 52240
Knoxville 50138

KANSAS
Leavenworth 66048
Topeka 66622
Wichita 67218

KENTUCKY
Lexington 40507
Louisville 40202

LOUISIANA
Alexandria 71301
New Orleans 70146
Shreveport 71130

MAINE
Togus 04330

MARYLAND
Baltimore 21218
Fort Howard 21052
Perry Point 21902

MASSACHUSETTS
Bedford 01730
Boston 02130
Brockton 02401
Northampton 01060
West Roxbury 02132

MICHIGAN
Allen Park 48101
Ann Arbor 48105
Battle Creek 49016
Iron Mountain 49801
Saginaw 48602

MINNESOTA
Minneapolis 55417
St. Cloud 56301

MISSISSIPPI
Biloxi 39531
Jackson 39216

MISSOURI
Columbia 65201
Kansas City 64128
Poplar Bluff 63901
St. Louis 63125

MONTANA
Fort Harrison 59636
Miles City 59301

NEBRASKA
Grand Island 68801
Lincoln 68510
Omaha 68105

NEVADA
Reno 89520

NEW HAMPSHIRE
Manchester 03104

NEW JERSEY
East Orange 07019
Lyons 07939

NEW MEXICO
Albuquerque 87108

NEW YORK
Albany 12208
Batavia 14020
Bath 14810
Bronx 10468
Brooklyn 11205
Buffalo 14215
Canandaigua 14424
Castle Point 12511
Montrose 10548
New York 10010
Northport (Long Island) 11768
Syracuse 13210

219

NORTH CAROLINA
Ashville 28805
Durham 27705
Fayetteville 28301
Salisbury 28144

NORTH DAKOTA
Fargo 58102

OHIO
Chillicothe 45601
Cincinnati 45220
Cleveland 44106
Dayton 45428

OKLAHOMA
Muskogee 74401
Oklahoma City 73104

OREGON
Portland 97207
Roseburg 97470

PENNSYLVANIA
Altoona 16603
Butler 16001
Coatesville 19320
Erie 16501
Lebanon 17042
Philadelphia 19104
Pittsburg (Highland Dr.) 15206
Pittsburgh (University Dr. C) 15240
Wilkes-Barre 18711

PUERTO RICO
San Juan 00936

RHODE ISLAND
Providence 02908

SOUTH CAROLINA
Charleston 29403
Columbia 29201

SOUTH DAKOTA
Fort Meade 57741
Hot Springs 57747
Sioux Falls 57101

TENNESSEE
Memphis 38104
Mountain Home
 (Johnson City) 37684
Murfreesboro 37130
Nashville 37203

TEXAS
Amarillo 79106
Big Spring 79720
Bonham 75418
Dallas 75216
*El Paso 79925
Houston 77211
Kerrville 78028
*Lubbock 79401
Marlin 76661
San Antonio
Temple 76501
Waco 76703

UTAH
Salt Lake City 84118

VERMONT
White River Junction 05001

VIRGINIA
Hampton 23667
Richmond 23249
Salem 24153

WASHINGTON
American Lake (Tacoma) 98493
Seattle 98108
Spokane 99208
Vancouver 98661
Walla Walla 99362

WEST VIRGINIA
Beckley 25801
Clarksburg 26301
Huntington 25704
Martinsburg 25401

WISCONSIN
Madison 53705
Tomah 54660
Wood (Milwaukee) 53193

WYOMING
Cheyenne 82001
Sheridan 82801

*Outpatient Clinic Only
**Domiciliary Only

Post-Certificate Programs

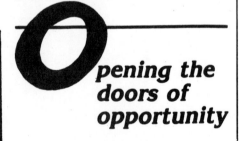

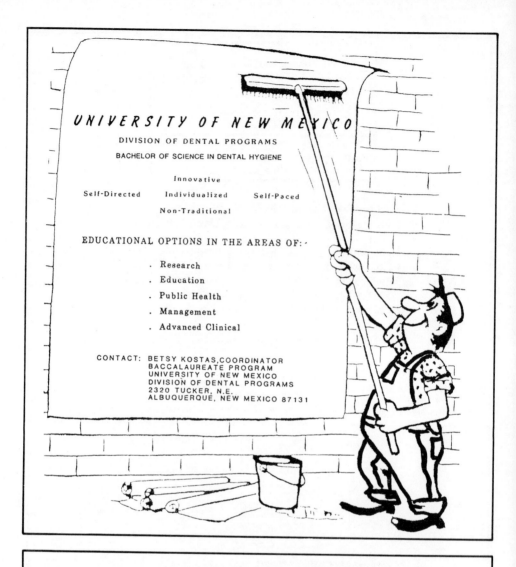

OLD DOMINION UNIVERSITY

A STANDARD OF EXCELLENCE
IN
DENTAL HYGIENE

DISTINGUISHED PROGRAMS
leading to the:

- Bachelor of Science Degree
  in Dental Hygiene
  (Entry Level and Degree
  Completion Programs)

- Master of Science Degree
  in Dental Hygiene

- Certificate in
  Dental Assisting

Curricula designed to
prepare graduates to assume
roles in:

- Research
- Oral Health Promotion
- Education
- Management/Administration
- Public Health
- Marketing
- Clinical Practice

Located in a major resort area with
easy access to Virginia Beach
and numerous historical, recreational
and cultural activities.

Coordinator, Degree Completion Program
School of Dental Hygiene and Dental Assisting
Old Dominion University
Norfolk, Virginia 23508
(804) 440-4310

Old Dominion University is an affirmative action, equal opportunity institution.

- -

For further information:

Name _____

Street _____

City, State, Zip _____

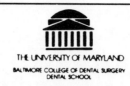
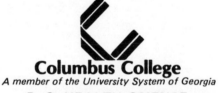

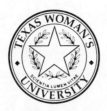
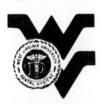

Medical University of South Carolina

College of Health Related Professions

Be it known that

_____?_____

having completed the prescribed course of study has been admitted

to the degree of

Bachelor of Science in Dental Hygiene

with all of the rights, privileges and responsibilities pertaining

to that degree

Does Your Name Belong on This?

. . . You May Be Closer Than You Think

* Post-certificate progression curriculum with emphasis in management, education and advanced clinical training;
* Primarily evening hours offerings with potential for dental hygiene employment opportunities and stipend;
* General education courses may be taken at your local college or university; and
* Part-time or full-time enrollment status.

For additional information, CONTACT: Professional Development Educational Department, Medical University of South Carolina, 171 Ashley Avenue, Charleston, SC 29425, (803) 792-3784.

REGINA DREYER THOMAS, RDH, BS, MPA

Ms. Dreyer brings with her a background of more than 25 years in the dental profession and industry. She has

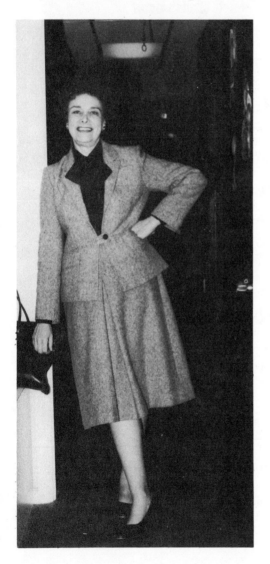

served as supervisor of a dental clinic in a large metropolitan hospital, been an assistant professor in a school of dental hygiene, a school dental hygienist, a registered dental hygienist and dental assistant in private practice, and a training director for a dental manufacturer.

Her present career centers around the dental industry as a training consultant for manufacturers and distributors. She is a consulting editor for *RDH* magazine, and publishes a variety of materials for dental health care professionals.

Her continuing education courses on career development and interpersonal skills are well attended by dental auxiliaries nationwide.